Laparoscopic Hysterectomy

To our patient wives, Judy and Elizabeth

Laparoscopic Hysterectomy

EDITED BY

RAY GARRY MD, FRCOG

Consultant Gynaecologist & Medical Director
The Women's Endoscopic Laser Foundation
South Cleveland Hospital, Middlesbrough, UK

AND

HARRY REICH MD, FACOG

Director of Gynecologic Surgery
Department of Gynecology
The Graduate Hospital
Philadelphia, Pennsylvania
and Nesbitt Memorial Hospital
Kingston, Pennsylvania

Provided as a service to medical education by
ZENECA Pharma International

The views expressed in this book
are not necessarily those of
ZENECA Pharma International

b

**Blackwell
Science**

© 1993 by
Blackwell Science Ltd
Editorial Offices:
Osney Mead, Oxford OX2 0EL
25 John Street, London WC1N 2BL
23 Ainslie Place, Edinburgh EH3 6AJ
238 Main Street, Cambridge
 Massachusetts 02142, USA
54 University Street, Carlton
 Victoria 3053, Australia

Other Editorial Offices:
Arnette Blackwell SA
 1, rue de Lille, 75007 Paris
 France

Blackwell Wissenschafts-Verlag GmbH
 Kurfürstendamm 57
 10707 Berlin, Germany

 Feldgasse 13, A-1238 Wien
 Austria

First published 1993
Reprinted 1994, 1995

Set by Setrite Typesetters, Hong Kong
Printed and bound in Great Britain
at the University Press, Cambridge

DISTRIBUTORS

Marston Book Services Ltd
PO Box 87
Oxford OX2 0DT
(*Orders*: Tel: 01865 791155
      Fax: 01865 791927
      Telex: 837515)

North America
 Blackwell Science, Inc.
 238 Main Street
 Cambridge, MA 02142
 (*Orders*: Tel: 800 215-1000
        617 876-7000
        Fax: 617 492-5263)
Australia
 Blackwell Science Pty Ltd
 54 University Street
 Carlton, Victoria 3053
 (*Orders*: Tel: 03 347-0300
        Fax: 03 349-3016)

A catalogue record for this title
is available from the British Library

ISBN 0-632-03465-3

Contents

List of Contributors

FAIZ HASHAM FFARCS
South Cleveland Hospital, Middlesbrough, UK

NICHOLAS KADAR MD, Grad IS
Director of Gynecologic Oncology and Endoscopic Surgery, Jersey Shore Medical Center, Neptune, New Jersey, USA

M.S. KOKRI FFARCS
South Cleveland Hospital, Middlesbrough, UK

THOMAS LYONS MD
Athens Women's Clinic, Athens, Georgia, USA

C.Y. LIU MD, FACOG
Director, Chattanooga Women's Laser Center, Chattanooga, Tennessee, USA

DOREEN MARTIN SRN
South Cleveland Hospital, Middlesbrough, UK

KURT SEMM FRCOG
Klinikum der Christian — Albrechts, Universität zu Kiel, Kiel, Germany

BEVERLEY SHALLOW SRN
South Cleveland Hospital, Middlesbrough, UK

Preface

The laparoscopic mode of access to abdominal surgery allows major intra-abdominal procedures to be performed without the need for large abdominal wounds. This permits less disfiguring and painful surgery to be achieved and also results in shortened postoperative recovery and convalescent times. Hysterectomy is one of the most commonly performed major surgical procedures and as more than 70% of all hysterectomies are still performed by the abdominal technique, the potential benefits for gynaecologists and their patients is considerable.

Laparoscopic hysterectomy is, however, a complex and technically difficult procedure, which requires considerable experience. Most gynaecologists are not yet familiar either with the equipment or the techniques needed for this type of surgery. To meet the need for detailed practical information about these procedures, we have brought together some of the world's most experienced gynaecological laparoscopists. This book is intended as a practical guide to complement workshops, didactic teaching and supervised preceptorships, to facilitate the safe introduction of these exciting techniques, which may be of great benefit to our patients.

R.G.
H.R.

1: Introduction

Hysterectomy is one of the most frequently performed of all surgical operations. The uterus traditionally has been removed by either the abdominal or the vaginal route. Between 1970 and 1978 more than 3 500 000 hysterectomies were performed in the US on women of reproductive age for non-malignant indications. Seventy-two per cent of these were performed using the abdominal approach. There is little evidence to suggest that this preference for abdominal hysterectomy is changing and in a recent study from a single centre in Scotland, of women under the age of 35 requiring a hysterectomy, 87.5% had the operation performed abdominally [1]. Even more striking is the evidence from a prospective study of 17 032 women reported in the Oxford—FPA study [2]. Over a period of 20 years, 1885 (11.1%) of those who enrolled in the study subsequently had a hysterectomy. Of this group of premenopausal women, only 224 (11.9%) had the operation performed vaginally. If those with a significant prolapse were excluded, then only 110 (6%) of premenopausal women coming to hysterectomy from 17 different centres in the UK had their hysterectomy vaginally. From this unique prospective study it would appear that almost 95% of women under 50 without major prolapse have their hysterectomy performed abdominally.

There has not always been this preference for the abdominal approach. The first hysterectomies attempted in modern times were vaginal. F.B. Osiander reported seven vaginal hysterectomies — all of whom died [3]. Subsequently, however, the German surgeon Conrad von Langenbeck performed the first successful vaginal hysterectomy for uterine cancer in 1815 [4]. This patient survived for 26 years. It was not until some 60 years later that the first successful abdominal hysterectomy was performed by W.A. Freund [5]. He introduced techniques for packing off the intestines, ligating the major blood-vessels, suturing the broad ligaments and closing the peritoneum. In spite of these technical advances, the mortality associated with this approach remained very high. T.G. Thomas reported in 1880 a death rate of 70% in a series of 365 abdominal hysterectomies [6].

Abdominal hysterectomy became the preferred operation following a series of surgical, anaesthetic and equipment advances. Several single-centre studies performed between 1940 and 1979 suggested that the morbidity at that time was greater after vaginal than abdominal hysterectomy. Premenopausal women who underwent vaginal hysterectomy appeared to suffer a particularly high morbidity. It was not until 1982 that Dicker et al. [7], in their careful multicentre study, presented evidence that the vaginal operation could be associated with a lower morbidity. The overall complication rate following abdominal hysterectomy was 70% higher than that following vaginal hysterectomy. Those who had abdominal hysterectomies had a longer stay in hospital and a more prolonged convalescent period. They also experienced more febrile morbidity and required more blood transfusions than those who had vaginal hysterectomies.

In the light of these findings it is interesting to speculate why such a high proportion of hysterectomies are still performed abdominally. Many gynaecologists find that vaginal hysterectomy is technically more difficult and correspondingly more dangerous in a younger woman with a well-supported uterus and some will only perform a vaginal hysterectomy when there is significant uterine prolapse. The need to inspect or remove the ovaries, fallopian tubes or other pelvic structures is, to most gynaecologists, a definite indication to remove the uterus abdominally. Fears of extensive endometriosis or pelvic adhesions are other contraindications to vaginal hysterectomy and yet such pathologies are among the most frequent indications for hysterectomy in the pre-menopausal woman.

The optimum approach to hysterectomy would be to retain the advantages of the abdominal route, which include clear visualization and ease of manipulation of the adnexal structures, and to combine these features with the principal advantage of vaginal hysterectomy, namely avoidance of a large abdominal incision. The use of laparoscopic techniques now permits this combined approach. The modern laparoscope gives a brilliant, magnified, two-dimensional image, which many consider superior to the view obtained at laparotomy. It and all the necessary ancillary instruments can be introduced through small stab incisions, avoiding long laparotomy scars. The laparoscopic approach can therefore combine excellent visualization of the pelvic structures with a minimum of abdominal wall scarring. This book discusses various ways in which the uterus and its adjacent structures can be mobilized and removed under full visual control without a laparotomy scar.

The purpose of this book is to discuss these new approaches to performing a hysterectomy. These new procedures add to the therapeutic options available to both patient and surgeon. In addition to the standard methods of abdominal and vaginal hysterectomy, there are now the methods of laparoscopic-assisted vaginal hysterectomy (LAVH), classic abdominal serrated macromorcellator hysterectomy (CASH) and full laparoscopic hysterectomy (LH). The relative importance of and indications for each of these techniques are not yet clear. It is, however, the authors' view that this minimally invasive approach to pelvic surgery offers many potential advantages both to the patient and to those providing health care. Endometriosis, fibroids and ovarian tumours are frequent indications for hysterectomy. Many women with these conditions can now have their lesions and their uterus removed without laparotomy scarring and the morbidity inevitably associated with it. With the use of advanced laparoscopic methods, even some forms of genital tract malignancy can be effectively managed laparoscopically. These advanced endoscopic techniques are not yet fully evaluated and the precise indications and contraindications for each approach have not yet been defined. They represent an important and perhaps major milestone in the development of our speciality. These are exciting times for the gynaecological surgeon and we feel privileged to have the opportunity to share in this book our enthusiasm for this new approach.

The considerable potential benefits to the patients and the health care providers amply justify the need to acquire new equipment and to develop new skills. It is hoped that this practically orientated book will be of value to those attempting to improve their skills in advanced operative laparoscopy and in particular to those wishing to become proficient in the techniques available to perform laparoscopic hysterectomy.

References

1 El Torkey MM. Hysterectomy in patients aged 35 years and under: indications and complications. *Obstet and Gynaecol Today* 1991; **1**: 44−49.
2 Vessey MP, Villard-Mackintosh L, McPherson K, Coulter A, Yeates D. The epidemiology of hysterectomy: findings in a large cohort study. *Br J Obstet Gynae* 1992; **99**: 402−407.
3 Osiander FB. Göttingen Gelerhte Anz. 1808; 130; 1861: 16.
4 Langenbeck CJA, Geschichte einer von MIR. Glücklich Verichteten Exstirpation der ganzer Gebärmutter. *N Biblioth, Chir Ophth* 1815; **1**: 551.
5 Freund WA. Zur einer Methode der totaler Uterus-Exstirpation. *Zbl Gyn* 1878; **12**: 265−269.
6 Mathiev A. The history of hysterectomy. *West J Surg Obstet Gynae* 1934; **42**: 1−13.
7 Dicker RG, Greenspan JR, Strauss LT, *et al.* Complications of abdominal and vaginal hysterectomy among women of reproductive age in the United States. *Am J Obstet Gynecol* 1982; **144**: 841−848.

2: The Development of Operative Gynaecological Laparoscopy

With the introduction of equipment that permits effective colposcopy, hysteroscopy, falloposcopy and laparoscopy, it is now possible to inspect every portion of the female genital tract in some considerable detail. Modern endoscopic optical equipment produces brilliant, detailed and magnified views of almost any aspect of pelvic pathology. Concomitant advances in conventional instrumentation and major developments in the fields of electronic and laser technology now allow a more precise and less invasive approach to treatment to be undertaken. To better understand the more important features of these highly developed modern endoscopic systems, it is useful to reflect on the difficulties our predecessors encountered in their attempts to visualize the internal structures and to study the solutions they found.

Endoscopic problems

Illumination

The origins of endoscopy can be traced to the Greek school of Kos led by Hippocrates (460–375 BC), who described the use of rectal and primitive vaginal specula. The Babylonian Talmud (500 AD) describes the use of a 'siphopherot', which was a lead tube that, when inserted into the vagina, permitted the cervix to be visualized. This is the first account in history of an internal organ being directly visualized.

The father of modern endoscopy was Bozinni, whose first attempt at endoscopy was to observe the interior of the urethra with a simple tube and a candle. He recognized that one of the essential requirements for any form of endoscopy was the need for adequate illumination. All internal body cavities are completely dark and, in order to be inspected, the structures require the transmission of adequate external illumination. Bozinni in 1860 [1] responded to this need by developing a light reflector, which was a rather complex system by which light from a lamp was reflected down a tube into the vagina for illumination whilst the operator observed the cervix through a second channel. The first truly practical endoscope was produced by Desmormeaux in Paris (1865) [2]. The method of illumination used was a lamp that burned a mixture of alcohol and turpentine. The endoscopic sleeve was a plain hollow tube attached to the light source (Fig. 2.1). Desmormeaux used this apparatus mainly for examination of the urethra and bladder. This equipment may indeed have been a significant conceptual advance in its time but that the technique was adopted says much for the fortitude

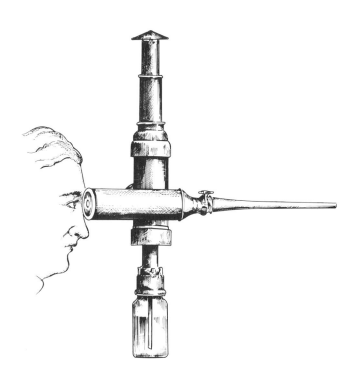

Fig. 2.1 The Desmormeaux endoscopic apparatus. Reproduced with permission from Baggish MS, Barbot J, Valle RF. *Diagnostic and Operative Hysteroscopy*: *A Text and Atlas*. Year Book Medical Publishers, Chicago.

of his patients who permitted an apparatus bellowing smoke and fumes to be inserted where man had been but never seen before. Pantaleoni in Ireland (1869) described using the endoscope of Desmormeaux to perform the first successful hysteroscopy when he demonstrated endometrial polyps to be the cause of postmenopausal bleeding [3].

Edison invented the incandescent light in 1880 and in 1883 Newman first described a superior endoscope using this more convenient source of light. The power of these incandescent light sources used to illuminate body cavities progressively increased. Unfortunately, the amount of heat produced also increased. The light source was held in or near the patient and local burns subsequently followed. In 1943 Fourestier, Gladu and Vulmière [4] overcame this problem by moving the light source some distance from the patient. They achieved this by transmitting light down a solid quartz rod. This advance considerably reduced the risk of local burns and electrical accidents. Such 'cold' light sources have subsequently been further improved by replacing the solid rod with bundles of flexible quartz fibres and more recently with 'liquid light' cables containing alcohol.

Optics

The Desmoreaux endoscope was a simple hollow tube with the tissue to be inspected at one end and the observer's eye at the other. Often little or nothing could be seen with this apparatus, especially if the tissue covered the end of the tube. Nitze (1879) [5] was the first to add a lens system to the endoscopic tube. This system not only protected the observer's eye but also improved visualization by magnifying the area being examined. These early lens systems were of poor quality and required very wide lenses and telescopes with a correspondingly large bore, frequently in excess of 12 mm diameter. Smaller, more precisely ground lenses were gradually developed, enabling smaller endoscopes to be produced without loss of optical resolution. In 1928 Kalk in Germany produced a much improved instrument with a new 135° lens system for oblique viewing. With better optics, the instruments became more widely used, particularly in continental Europe. In 1952 Hopkins and Kapany in Reading, UK, developed the Rod-Lens system. This gives both a brighter image and better definition. In a standard endoscope there is an eyepiece, an objective lens system and a number of relay lenses encased in a rigid tube. These lenses are thin and are separated by relatively long air-filled spaces. In the Hopkins rod-lens system the lenses are elongated and almost fill the tube with only short airspaces between (Fig. 2.2). Filling the space between objective and eyepiece with glass rather than air more than doubles the transmission of light. In addition, light transmission through an endoscope is proportional to the fourth power of the internal aperture radius and the rod-lens system allows a 1.4 times larger internal radius for a given outer radius. Thus the combined increase in light transmission of the rod-lens system over thin-lens relay is around nine times.

Pneumatoperitoneum

In addition to the optical and illumination problems inherent in all forms of endoscopy, visualization of the abdominal cavity presents several unique difficulties. The first examination of the abdominal contents of a living animal was described by Dr Georg Kelling to the German Biological and Medical Society in 1902 [6]. He termed the examination celioscopy. He appreciated that the view was dramatically improved when he created a pneumatoperitoneum by forcing air filtered through cotton wool into the cavity. This preliminary step both reduced the risks of damaging the abdominal contents during insertion of the

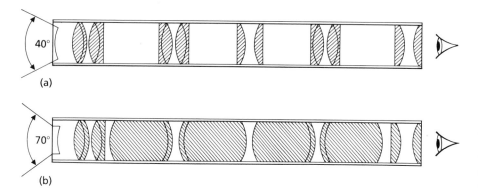

Fig. 2.2 The Hopkins rod-lens system. Reproduced with permission from Baggish MS, Barbot J, Valle RF. *Diagnostic and Operative Hysteroscopy: A Text and Atlas*. Year Book Medical Publishers, Chicago.

endoscope and prevented loops of bowel obscuring vision. Jacobeus of Stockholm first described the inspection of the peritoneal cavity in humans and he was the first to use the term laparoscopy in 1910 [7]. He did not in fact develop a pneumatoperitoneum but his success may have been due to the fact that he restricted his investigations to patients with ascites. Nordentoeft in 1912 improved laparoscopy by facilitating the insertion of the telescope with a trocar system [8].

Once the value of a pneumatoperitoneum became established, the next problem was how this could be safely established. Special needles were developed to minimize the risk of penetrating intra-abdominal structures. The first of these was invented by Goetze (1918) [9] and this design was improved on by Janos Veress of Hungary [10] (Fig. 2.3).

A major hazard in insufflating gas into the peritoneal cavity is the risk of venous air embolism. There is no physiological mechanism to transport nitrogen but quite large quantities of carbon dioxide can be carried and metabolized by physiological mechanisms. The substitution of CO_2 for air was first suggested by Zollikofer in Switzerland (1924) [11]. Even with this much safer gas, fatal venous air embolism remains a risk of laparoscopy. It was appreciated that careful control of the intra-abdominal pressure during insufflation greatly reduced this risk. In the early 1950s Frangenheim in Konstanz made the first prototype of an automatic infusion apparatus [12]. Semm, from Kiel, developed a completely automatic, pressure-controlled system to set and limit the pressure produced in the cavity during insufflation [13].

Palmer in France pioneered the post-war development of diagnostic laparoscopy, particularly for the investigation of infertility [14]. He and Te Linde in the US briefly tried the transvaginal culdoscopic approach to endoscopy but soon reverted to laparoscopy because it gave a better view of the pelvis. Palmer also developed many ancillary instruments for the diagnostic and surgical treatment of gynaecological disorders.

Operative laparoscopy

With good visualization and a safe, well-maintained pneumatoperitoneum, it became clear that laparoscopy could be used for therapy as

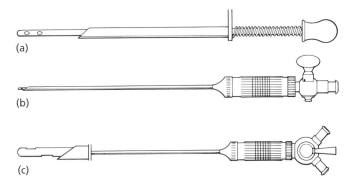

Fig. 2.3 Various early safety needles for inducing a pneumatoperitoneum. (a) Goetze insufflation needle; (b) Veress modification; (c) Semm modification. Reproduced with permission from Sanfilippo JS, Levine RC (eds) *Operative Gynecologic Endoscopy*. Springer-Verlag, New York, 1989.

well as diagnosis. The first reported operative laparoscopic procedure was that performed by Fevers in 1933 [15]. He was a general surgeon who performed an abdominal adhesiolysis. In 1937 Ruddock introduced a drill biopsy forceps with diathermy coagulation potential [16]. Perhaps the first gynaecological operative laparoscopy was performed by Boesch in Switzerland in 1936 [17], although an American surgeon, E.T. Anderson, appeared to independently suggest that an electrical coagulation system could be used as a method of female sterilization [18]. Power and Barnes were the first to describe a series of sterilizations, performed in 1941, in which, using Ruddock's equipment, they fulgurated a 1-cm portion of the cornual section of each tube [19]. This technique became the most commonly used method of sterilization for the next 30 years.

Electrosurgery using unipolar diathermy in this manner involves the transmission of electrical energy from the electrode point inside the abdomen through the tissues to a large receiving electrode on the patient's skin. Using such unipolar circuitry to coagulate tubes produced some burns, the cause of which was poorly understood at the time. These led to infection, peritonitis and deaths from bowel perforations and to avoid this complication Frangenheim [20] in Germany and Rioux and Cloutier [21] in Canada introduced bipolar diathermy. These techniques were subsequently popularized as a method of tubal sterilization by Kleppinger and Corson. With this technique, current flows only between the two electrodes, which are usually the blades of the tissue forceps.

Kurt Semm, with typical flair, adopted a different approach to the prevention of electrical burns. He developed a laparoscopic modification of his endocoagulator. With this system, electrical energy is used to heat the tip of the coagulator probe to a controlled temperature of 100°C. Biological tissues will be coagulated by the heat generated but without coming into contact with any electrical current.

Lasers

The CO_2 laser was introduced into laparoscopic surgery by Bruhat and his group in Clermont-Ferrand in 1979 [22]. This laser, with its precise cutting ability, has been widely used to divide adhesions and cut tissue. This laser wavelength cannot easily be transmitted down a flexible fibre and must instead be reflected to the tissues by a series of mirrors which are somewhat bulky and cumbersome. The other disadvantage of this wavelength is that it acts by heating cells to 100°C and boiling the intracellular water. This rapid vaporization of tissues produces large quantities of smoke and water vapour, which can obscure vision. Various techniques have been developed to minimize these disadvantages and these will be discussed fully in subsequent chapters.

Another approach to overcoming these problems has been to use other laser wavelengths, particularly the neodymium-doped yttrium—aluminium—garnet (Nd-YAG), potassium-titanyl-phosphate (KTP) and argon bands, to cut and coagulate tissues. Each of these laser wavelengths can be transmitted down a flexible quartz fibre and this is often more convenient in day-to-day use than the CO_2 laser. Each of the fibre lasers produces less smoke and a greater coagulation and haemostatic effect than the CO_2 laser and these properties are utilized clinically. However, they produce a less precise cutting effect with a greater degree of lateral thermal damage and consequent greater risk of unintended tissue damage.

Good techniques in laparoscopic surgery seek to mimic the techniques which would be employed in open surgery. In all types of surgery, the first principle is to ensure good access and exposure of the tissues to be removed. In open surgery, this requires the correct placement of an adequate-sized incision. In laparoscopy, it requires the insertion, through a small periumbilical incision, of an excellent optical system linked to a good light source and visual system. To ensure optimum vision, the abdomen must also be distended to a safe pressure and a pneumatoperitoneum continuously maintained.

At open surgery, tissues must be handled gently, trauma from packing and handling minimized and peritoneal surfaces kept moist. During laparoscopic surgery, there are no tissue 'handling', minimal tissue disturbance and no packing, and the corresponding trauma to peritoneal surfaces is avoided. The abdominal cavity remains essentially closed and there is very little opportunity for serosal drying.

At open surgery, tissues to be removed are freed by sharp and blunt dissection, using knife, scissors, pressure and counter-traction. Diathermy and lasers are also occasionally used. Each of these modalities is used in a modified form laparoscopically but, because of the constraints of the approach, each modality is often delivered more precisely during endoscopic surgery.

Adequate haemostasis is essential for optimum surgery. The traditional methods for open surgery of suture and diathermy have been complemented by clips, staples and lasers. Ingenious modifications of existing technology and some exciting new devices mean that all of these options are now also available for laparoscopic surgery.

In summary, the benefits of avoiding large skin incisions are becoming increasingly apparent. Good clinical results will follow when the time-tested principles of open surgery are applied to the laparoscopic approach. This chapter summarizes the contributions of some of the many innovative pioneers who have brought us to the situation where operations such as laparoscopic hysterectomy can be performed with safety and with the possibility of better clinical outcomes than can be achieved with classical surgery.

References

1 Bozinni P. Der Lichtleiter oder Beschreibung einer einfachen Vorrichtung und Anwendung zur erleuchtung innerer Höhler und Zwischenräume des Lebenden animalischen Körpers. Weimar, Landes-Industrie-Comptoir, 1807.

2 Desmormeaux AJ. Transactions of the Société de Chirurgie, Paris. *Gazette des Hop* 1865.

3 Pantaleoni D. On endoscopic examination of the cavity of the womb. *Med Press Circ* 1869; **8**: 26.

4 Fourestier M, Gladu A, Vulmière J. La peritoneoscopie. *Presse Médicale* 1943; **5**: 46–47.

5 Nitze H. Über eine neue Behandlungsmethode der Höhlen des menschlichen Körpers. *Wein Med Wochenschr* 1879; **24**: 851–858.

6 Kelling G. Über Oesophagoskopie, Gastroskopie und Colioskopie. *Münchener Wochenschrift* 1902; **49**: 21–24.

7 Jacobeus HC. Über die Möglichkeit, die Zystoskopie bei Untersuchung seröser Höhlungen anzuwenden. *Münch Med Wochenschr* 1910; **57**: 2090–2092.

8 Nordentoeft S. Über endoskopie geschlosener Kavitäten mittels eines Trokarendoskopes. *Verhandlungen der Deutschen Gesellschaft für Gynäkologie* 1912; **41**: 78–81.

9 Goetze O. Die Röntgendiagnostik bei gasgetfullter Bauchole — eine neue Methode. *Münch Med Wochenschr* 1918; **65**: 1275–1280.

10 Veress J. Ein neues Instrument zur Ausführung von Brust — oder Bauchpunktionen und Pneumothoraxbehandlung. *Deutsche Med Wochenschr* 1938; **64**: 1480–1481.

11 Zollikofer R. Zur Laparoskopie. *Schweizerische Med Wochenschr* 1924; **5**: 264–265.

12 Frangenheim H. *Die Laparoskopie und die Kulposkopie in der Gynäkologie.* Thieme, Stuttgart, 1959.

13 Semm K. Die kontrollierte und dosierbare Wärmekoagulation der gutachtigen, portio veränderung Geburtshilfe. *Frauenheilkd* 1965; **25**: 795–802.

14 Palmer R. Gynecologic celioscopy: report of Prof MacQuot. *Acad Chir* 1946; **76**: 363–368.

15 Fevers C. Die Laparoskopie mit dem Cystoskope. Ein Beitrag zur Vereinfachung der Technik und zur endoskopischen Strangdurchtrennung in der Bauchhöhlele. *Med Klinik* 1933; **29**: 1042–1045.

16 Ruddock JC. Peritoneoscopy. *Surg Gynaecol Obstet* 1937; **65**: 623.

17 Boesch PF. Laparoskopie. *Schweiz z. Krankenhaus Anstaltsw* 1936; **6**: 62.

18 Anderson ET. Peritoneoscopy. *Am J Surg* 1937; **35**: 136–139.

19 Power FH, Barnes AC. Sterilization by means of peritoneoscopic fulguration: a preliminary report. *Am J Obstet Gynaecol* 1941; **41**: 1038–1043.

20 Frangenheim H. *Laparoscopy and Culposcopy in Gynaecology.* Butterworths, London, 1972.

21 Rioux JE, Cloutier D. Bipolar cautery for sterilization by laparoscopy. *J Repro Med* 1974; **13**: 6–10.

22 Bruhat MA, Mage G, Nanhes H. Use of the CO_2 laser by laparoscopy. In: Kaplan I (ed.) *Laser Surgery III.* Proceedings of the Third International Congress on Laser Surgery, pp. 275–281. Jerusalem Press, Tel Aviv, 1979.

3: Instrumentation for Laparoscopic Surgery

Pneumatoperitoneum

Distension gas

The vast majority of gynaecologists consider it essential to establish an adequate pneumatoperitoneum before inserting the primary trocar. A minority consider that, if the abdominal wall is lifted away from the abdominal contents and the trocar is directed at the correct angle, the primary trocar may be inserted prior to the induction of the pneumatoperitoneum. The advantage of this latter approach is that the laparoscopic cannula is of much larger diameter than the Veress needle and the abdomen can therefore be distended much more rapidly. In general, this approach demands greater skill and sureness of touch and should not be attempted unless highly skilled and can then probably only be justified in cases where speed is of the essence.

Air, nitrogen and carbon dioxide have been used to produce abdominal distension at laparoscopy. The main risk associated with the production of a pneumatoperitoneum is that the gas under pressure will be forced into a vein and produce a venous air embolism. Such gas will rapidly accumulate in the right side of the heart and produce bubbles which render cardiac activity ineffective in pumping blood around the body. The risk of such an embolism is inversely related to the solubility of the gas used. Nitrous oxide is 30 times more soluble than nitrogen but is only 68% as soluble as carbon dioxide in blood. There are elaborate physiological mechanisms which can transport significant quantities of CO_2 in the blood in soluble form. It is estimated that some 150 ml/min of CO_2 can be transported in this way. Since carbon dioxide is the most soluble of the gases available, it is the gas associated with the lowest risk of air embolism. The capacity of these physiological mechanisms, however, is limited and can be overwhelmed. More complex laparoscopic procedures demand longer operating times and modern equipment has the potential to pump in many litres of gas every minute. It is therefore essential to ensure that the infused gas freely enters the cavity and does not go directly into an open vein. Both the rate of flow of the gas and the pressure of gas in the abdominal cavity should be carefully controlled. Nitrous oxide is a flammable gas and can support combustion and there is a definite risk of an intra-abdominal explosion, especially if electrosurgical instruments or lasers are also used. In contrast, carbon dioxide is an inert gas and can be used with such equipment without the risk of an intra-abdominal conflagration.

Carbon dioxide is produced commercially in large quantities, is readily available and is cheap. It is almost certainly the safest gas available. It does, however, possess undesirable properties. This soluble gas can dissolve in peritoneal fluid and form carbonic acid. This acid irritates the peritoneum and the diaphragm and may account for the characteristic abdominal and shoulder tip discomfort felt after any laparoscopy. Carbon dioxide can also produce both a metabolic and a respiratory acidosis, manifested by a reduction in arterial pH. Cardiac arrhythmias are common and have been reported in 27% of all laparoscopic procedures. The most common changes are sinus tachycardia, ventricular arrhythmias and asystole. These arrhythmias may be due to the elevated carbon dioxide levels in the blood but are more likely to be related to excessive vasovagal reflexes produced by peritoneal stimulation and to hypoxia. This subject is discussed in more detail in Chapter 9.

Recommendation

Carbon dioxide is the insufflation gas of choice but its metabolic and cardiac effects must be carefully monitored.

Insufflation

Gas will only flow into the peritoneal cavity under pressure. The higher the pressure, the greater the risk of the gas being forced into the circulation and producing a venous embolism. It is important to monitor and restrict the abdominal pressure to the lowest level compatible with optimum operating conditions. A pressure of 10−15 mmHg is usually adequate and should only be exceeded in specific circumstances. In addition to the risk of venous embolism, pressures above this level may also compress the vena cava and reduce the venous return to the heart.

Reich recommends that, after ensuring a steady state, the abdominal pressure be deliberately increased to 25 mmHg immediately prior to the insertion of the primary trocar. This high pressure ensures that the abdominal wall is drum-tight, facilitating the easy and safe insertion of the trocars. If this technique is chosen, it is essential that the abdominal pressure is reduced to 10−15 mmHg as soon as trocar insertion is complete.

Once established, it is important to maintain an adequate pneumatoperitoneum. Care must be taken to ensure that both the volume and the pressure of the gas in the abdomen are controlled. Modern electronically controlled apparatus permits a predetermined pressure level to be selected and the flow of gas to be automatically adjusted to maintain this preselected level (Figs 3.1−3.3).

The use of multiple puncture sites and the frequent withdrawal and

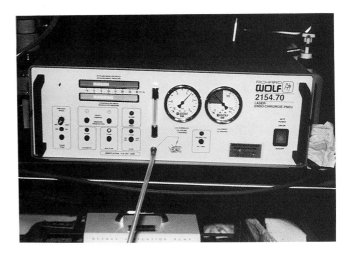

Fig. 3.1 Wolf electronically controlled insufflator.

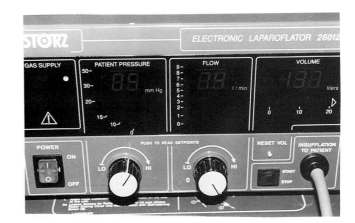

Fig. 3.2 Storz electronic laparoflator.

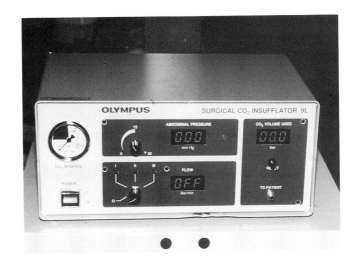

Fig. 3.3 Olympus surgical insufflator.

reinsertion of instruments often results in loss of gas during a complex procedure. This loss can be minimized with good technique and by using well-designed trocars with effective gas traps. Only relatively small quantities of gas should be lost in this way and with modern equipment this should seldom lead to impairment of vision. Gas can be lost very rapidly if the trocar sheath is inadvertently withdrawn with the instrument but this can be prevented by good trocar design. An inescapable cause of rapid loss of gas, however, is during rapid abdominal suction aspiration to remove fluid and blood from the cavity. Large quantities of gas will inevitably be removed during such a manoeuvre and, as this is often performed at a critical or even dangerous time in the operation, it is important that vision is not then lost. Large volumes of gas may be deliberately vented when vision is obscured by smoke and plume. To replace large volumes of CO_2 rapidly, insufflators of ever-increasing flow rates are being introduced. Early laparoscopic insufflators had a maximum flow rate of 3 litres/min but more recently introduced models have capacities of 9, 12, 16 or even 32 litres/min. We are concerned that very high flow rates may be used simply to cover poor technique and may result in an increased risk of venous air embolism, but in specific circumstances a fast flow rate of CO_2 is most useful. We have found flow rates around 9 litres/ min adequate for most circumstances.

In most early laparoscopic insufflators the external bottle of pressurized CO_2 fed the insufflator's small-capacity internal tank. Most gynaecological theatres still use such equipment. The capacity of these internal tanks is 10—12 litres, which is only appropriate for the very shortest of diagnostic procedures. Such apparatus is totally unsuitable for prolonged and complex laparoscopic surgery, as the gas supply will last for only a few minutes before vision is lost. The procedure will then have to be interrupted to allow the internal tank to be refilled and vision to be restored. This is time-consuming, irritating and potentially dangerous. For advanced laparoscopic procedures it is essential to be able to take the gas directly from a large, high-pressure, external gas cylinder.

The insufflator should have simple displays to indicate the intra-abdominal pressure and the gas flow rates continuously. The pressure may be inadvertently raised:
1   during the insertion of the trocars;
2   when the patient is straining if anaesthesia is light;
3   with excessive gas flow from a source extrinsic to the insufflator, e.g. when using an Nd-YAG laser with a CO_2-cooled sapphire tip;
4   if the gas line from the insufflator becomes blocked or kinked;
5   if the insufflation needle has failed to enter the cavity and lies in the abdominal wall.

The use of diathermy or laser in the abdomen may create smoke and plume which can impair vision. Several modern insufflators incorporate a closed-circuit system in which a second gas line leads from a trocar side-arm back to the insufflator. The contaminated gas is led through a filter to be cleaned and then led back to the abdominal cavity. It is hoped that such a system will avoid the need for frequent purging of the abdominal-cavity gases. It is claimed that such systems can provide continuous, clear, operating conditions and reduce the amount of CO_2 required during a procedure, but in our experience to date this has proved a little disappointing.

Recommendation

A modern, electronic, high-flow insufflator, with facilities for monitoring and automatically controlling the rate of gas flow and the intra-abdominal pressure, is recommended. It is important that the CO_2 is taken from a high-pressure, large-capacity, storage tank.

Visualization

In endoscopic surgery the quality of the surgery is dependent on the quality of the visual image. For the best results it is necessary to have a suitable and balanced combination of laparoscope, light source, light cable, video-camera and video-monitors. These components interact and the quality of the final image depends on the balance achieved between them. For example, as the 'chip' inside each generation of video-cameras increases in sensitivity, so the need for ever brighter light sources diminishes. It is not necessary to have the most sensitive camera in the world connected to the most powerful light source in the world via the most efficient light cable. Such a system may only achieve an overexposed 'white-out' image produced at very great cost. What is required is a carefully matched system which balances light output and transmission with camera sensitivity and monitor resolution.

Light generators

The quality of the light delivered to the endoscope depends on both the generator and the light cable. The simplest cold-light generators provide 150 watts of power (Fig. 3.4). Such systems are available in every operating room. They are compact, economical and effective for simple diagnostic procedures viewed directly down the endoscope. In advanced operative procedures it is essential to be able to obtain a panoramic view of the operating field and, if a video-camera is used, more powerful light sources are required. These systems use halogen and other metal halides as the primary light source, and a power of 300–400 W is now routinely available. The most powerful and effective light in general use is the 300 W xenon source (Fig. 3.5).

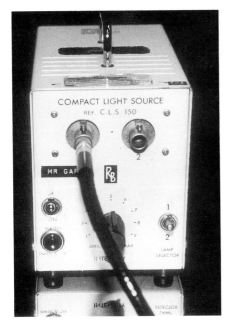

Fig. 3.4 Simple 150-watt light source similar to that found in all operating rooms. This type is inadequate for operative laparoscopy.

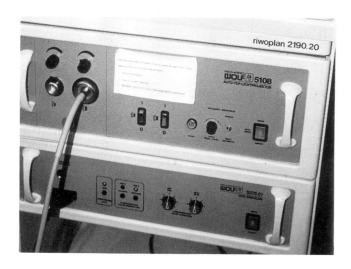

Fig. 3.5 Powerful 300–400-watt automatic halide light source of type suitable for operative light source.

Light cables

Increasing the number of optical fibres in an endoscope increases both the diameter of the scope and the quality of the image. Similarly, increasing the number of optical fibres and the thickness of the cable connecting the light source to the laparoscope can significantly increase the amount of transmitted light available. A marked improvement in optical quality can sometimes be achieved by simply replacing a standard-diameter 3.5-mm fibre with a 4.8- or 6-mm fibreoptic cable (Fig. 3.6). These quartz fibres fracture with wear and tear and should be checked frequently. Broken strands show up as black spots at the distal end of the illuminated fibre. If more than 20% of the fibre is blackened, the cable should be replaced. Cables filled with liquid alcohol transmit light somewhat more effectively than fibreoptic cables.

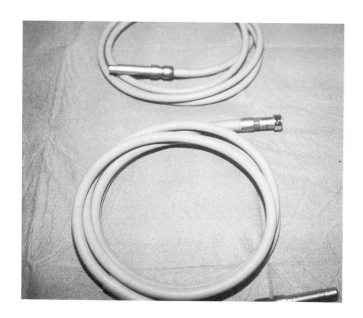

Fig. 3.6 3.5- and 4.8-mm fibreoptic light cables. Substituting the larger diameter cable can significantly increase the amount of light available in the abdomen.

These 'liquid-light' cables are heavily clad to prevent rupture and tend to be a little less flexible than a fibreoptic cable of similar diameter. The light they transmit is of a different colour and the equipment must be balanced accordingly.

Recommendation

A high-powered, xenon or similar, automatic, light source used in conjunction with a 4–6-mm fibreoptic or liquid-light cable in good condition should be used for optimum visualization.

Video-cameras

A video-camera and monitor are not luxuries but essential equipment for complex laparoscopic surgery, which may last for 2 or more hours. The surgeon cannot operate effectively and efficiently if he/she is bent in an uncomfortable position for long periods of time. In contrast, with good-quality video-pictures he/she can operate in an optimum position and can be assisted by the whole operating-theatre team. These video systems also provide unequalled opportunities for teaching and precise electronic documentation of the procedure (Fig. 3.7).

The introduction of the charge-coupled device (CCD), 'chip' by Boyle and Smith (1970) represents a further milestone in the evolution of advanced laparoscopic surgery. These CCD cameras are the third generation of endoscopic cameras. The previous generation of cameras gave good image quality but were heavy, unwieldy and unsuitable for fine manipulation. The silicon chip permitted the development of much

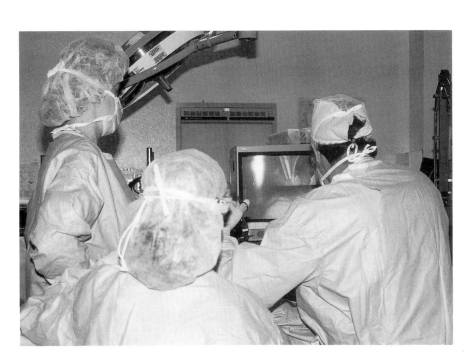

Fig. 3.7 The surgeon and his team operating and assisting in optimum conditions.

smaller, lightweight cameras capable of giving superb visual images (Fig. 3.8). A 'chip' consists of a large number of photocell receptors tightly packed together in a grid. Each receptor depends on the sensitivity of silicon to light. Light striking a silicon receptor decreases the electrical resistance of the silicon and generates current. Each silicon receptor generates one pixel, which is the smallest unit of the picture elements of an image. The number of pixels that can fit on a chip determines the resolution of that chip. The average chip used in solid-state cameras today contains between 150 000 and 300 000 pixels. This corresponds to 450 horizontal lines per inch of resolution. The way the electrical charges are moved on the chip is called charge-coupling. Colour is identified by different red, green and blue pixels. To improve picture quality still further, a range of three-chip cameras has been introduced. This type of camera contains three separate chips, giving an increased picture resolution. In the PAL format, such a camera has 1 369 998 pixels, corresponding to 700 horizontal lines per inch. These cameras, however, are at present a little more difficult to set up and more expensive than the single-chip camera. It is doubtful that at this

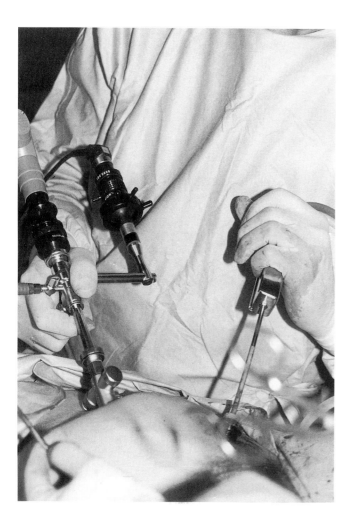

Fig. 3.8 A lightweight CCD camera attached to an operating laparoscope.

time the three-chip camera offers sufficient advantage over the already excellent picture quality obtained from some single-chip systems to justify the extra cost. A development eagerly awaited, however, is the introduction of three-dimensional video systems and other 'virtual-reality' and 'telepresence' systems, which are being developed to increase the realism and true-to-laparotomy feel of the systems used.

Most cameras have a function to enable them to be 'white-balanced'. Before use, the camera is directed at a pure white background and colour balancing is automatically performed to reset the image to absolute white. This ensures an accurate spectrum of colours for the procedure and, as the subtle colour differences may be essential in some dissections etc., it is important that this is done before each session. Most cameras now also have a means for both automatically and manually varying the light intensity during use. The auto function measures the available light and then automatically adjusts the diameter of the iris. All cameras must obviously have a focusing device, and some have a zoom facility. We have not found this latter, expensive feature of significant value.

Recommendation

There are so many excellent video systems available that it is impossible to make specific recommendations. It is important to use a balance system with a single-chip CCD camera with automatic iris control.

Video monitors

The camera is an optical—electronic interface when attached to the endoscope. A cable transmits this electronic impulse to a control unit, which processes and then transmits the image to the video-monitor. This camera control unit is usually mounted near the video-monitors.

All the members of the operating team depend on the quality of the image and it is important that the resolution of the monitors is of a high enough standard to take advantage of the quality of the image generated by the CCD cameras. A standard monitor has a resolution of 400 horizontal lines, but superior picture resolution will be obtained with a 700-line monitor. As with a domestic audio system where the quality of the sound obtained is determined by the quality of the weakest link in the turntable, pick-up, amplifier and speaker chain, so with an operating video system expensive cameras, light sources and laparoscopes will be found to be inadequate unless monitors with the highest possible resolution are also used. For maximum comfort and visibility it is advisable to use two monitors, one on each side of the patient. The monitors should be positioned so that the surgeon and his/her assistants both have an image in direct line of site and the monitor screen size should be at least 13 inches in size for adequate visibility. We currently use two Sony 48-cm Trinitron monitors, which have 700 horizontal lines' resolution.

Recommendation

A pair of large, 700 horizontal lines' resolution monitors will give the best possible visualization.

Laparoscopes

As discussed in Chapter 2, the Hopkins rod-lens system produces superior images and should always be used for rigid-telescope endoscopy. For pelvic endoscopic surgery, it is particularly important to achieve a large panoramic view to enable a correct perspective to be maintained. It is also important to have a wide depth of focus so that clear, highly magnified, close-up views can also be obtained.

Most authorities prefer a 0°, forward-viewing scope, which gives the surgeon a natural perspective (Fig. 3.9). Occasionally a 30° forward-oblique scope can be helpful to visualize partially obscured areas. The quality of the image is related to the size of the telescope and in most circumstances a 10-mm scope inserted through the umbilical portal is preferred. If a laser is to be used, a smaller 5-mm telescope mounted alongside a 5-mm operating channel is frequently preferred (Fig. 3.10). This smaller optical pathway inevitably compromises the brightness of the image but with an otherwise optimum system the image can still be satisfactory. Operating laparoscopes require the optic pathway to be offset and this can be achieved with either an angled or a crankshaft design (Figs 3.11 and 3.12).

Recommendation

Use a 0°, Hopkins rod-lens, rigid laparoscope with a 10-mm telescope unless an in-line operating function is required.

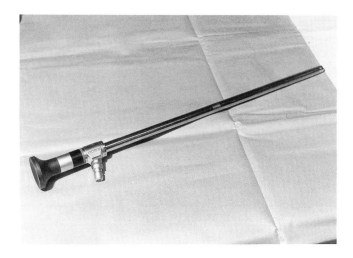

Fig. 3.9 A 10-mm 0° laparoscope.

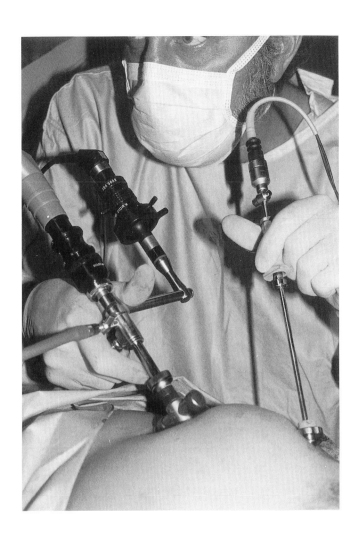

Fig. 3.10 An operating laparoscope connected to a CO_2 laser and a video-camera.

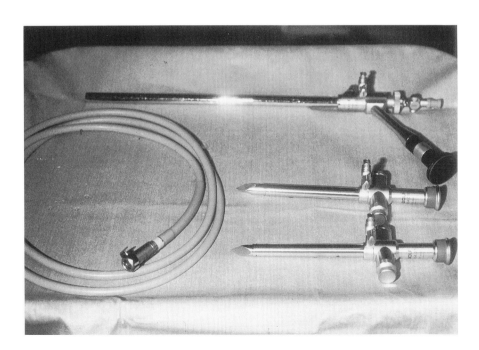

Fig. 3.11 An operating laparoscope with angled optics.

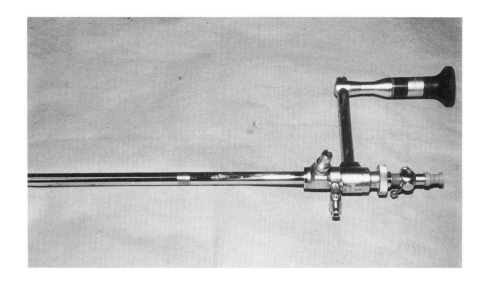

Fig. 3.12 An operating laparoscope with crankshaft optic.

Fogging

The image quality can be impaired by 'fogging' or condensation on any of the optical glass interfaces. This most commonly occurs between the telescope optic lens and the outer surface of the video-camera lens. Condensation occurs when moist, relatively warm air comes into contact with cooler glass surfaces. This often occurs if the scope or the camera has been stored at a lower temperature outside the operating room and is returned immediately before use. Soaking the camera for disinfection increases the risk of droplets of moisture becoming trapped between the lens surfaces. To avoid these problems we store all cameras and optical equipment at the same even temperature as the operating room and we no longer immerse the scope in fluid at any time. Disinfection of the camera is restricted to wiping the external surfaces with an alcohol-soaked swab and ensuring that every surface is completely dry before use.

If, in spite of these precautions, fogging still occurs, it can be managed by exposing the affected surfaces to air, drying the glass thoroughly and then applying an antifogging agent. We have found FRED (fog reduction and elimination device obtainable from Dexide Ltd) effective for this purpose. Other solutions, involving modifications to the design of the camera–telescope interface, have been introduced. Circon (ACMI, Stamford, CT) have produced a ventilated laparoscope interface and claim that the air flow will eliminate this problem of fogging. The ultimate but most expensive answer to this problem is to connect the camera permanently and directly to the laparoscope.

If the distal end of the laparoscope optic becomes obscured with blood or debris, vision is obviously impaired. It can often be cleaned by wiping the lens on the peritoneum (the 'peritoneal handkerchief'). If this is ineffective, spraying fluid from the irrigation cannula in the manner of a 'windscreen washer' will usually restore crystal-clear vision.

Circon have introduced a telescope with a similar but in-built irrigation system to keep the lens clear. These measures sometimes fail and it may be necessary to remove the scope and wipe the end with detergent or FRED.

Recommendation

To prevent fogging keep all optical and camera equipment completely dry and at a constant temperature.

Pneumatoperitoneum needles

An inherent risk of laparoscopy is that the needle used to establish the initial pneumatoperitoneum might inadvertently penetrate an important abdominal structure. Special needles have been designed to minimize but not completely eliminate this danger. That designed by Veress remains the most commonly used. It is made up of an outer cannula with a bevel cutting edge, inside which is a spring-loaded, central, gas-carrying tube. The central hollow tube has distal perforations and is connected via a luer lock at its proximal end to the infusion gas line. When the needle is advanced through the various layers of the abdominal wall, the central, round-ended column is forced back inside the cannula, exposing the sharp cutting edge. This passes easily through the subcutaneous tissues. As soon as the tip enters the cavity the resistance on the probe is released and it again comes to protrude beyond the sharp cutting edge, thereby protecting the abdominal structures from inadvertent perforation. Fine, sharp, disposable needles are now available, which are very easy to introduce but, because of their narrow diameter, result in slower insufflation.

Recommendation

A sharp Veress needle remains the optimum needle to induce a pneumatoperitoneum.

Trocars

Sharp trocars and their associated sheaths are required to permit the introduction of instruments into the abdominal cavity. The smallest size required to accommodate all the instruments to be used in that particular portal should be chosen. The most frequently used sizes are 5 mm and 10 mm (Fig. 3.13). If different-diameter instruments are to be inserted, a size suitable for the largest instrument must be selected and the working diameter reduced when appropriate by using reducing sleeves or caps.

The sharp point of the trocar may be either pyramidal or conical in

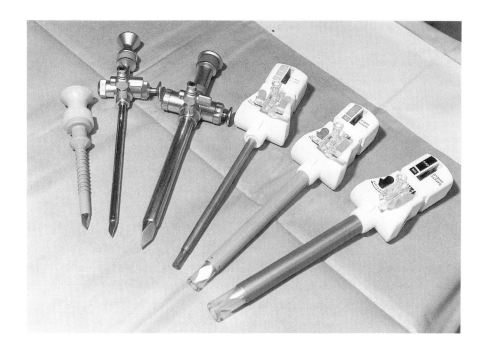

Fig. 3.13 A variety of trocars and sheaths.

shape and there remains a difference in opinion as to the better design. Those who favour the smoother conical shape believe that it is less traumatic as this shape is less likely to damage blood-vessels because it will push them out of the way rather than severing them. It is claimed that this shape is therefore less likely to produce a haematoma in the abdominal wall. Pyramidal-shaped trocars have sharp cutting edges and proponents believe that they are easier to insert through tough fascial layers. Unintended trauma to the abdominal contents is more likely to occur when extra force is required to insert a relatively blunt trocar through resisting tissues. This is less likely to occur with pyramidal-shaped tips and for this reason this shape is preferred by the authors.

The introduction of disposable trocars by Ethicon Endosurgery (Cincinnati, OH) and USSC (Norwalk, CT) may make this controversy irrelevant for, if the considerable extra costs can be accommodated, then it is possible to ensure a perfectly sharp trocar every time. These disposable devices also have a safety shield of plastic covering the trocar point. These spring-loaded devices cover the point of the trocar at all times except when being inserted through the abdominal wall. It is claimed that this will substantially reduce the risks of damage to the underlying structures.

A major problem with trocar design is to ensure that the sheath stays secured in the correct position for the duration of the procedure. The older reusable sheaths are relatively long and with an outer surface of smooth metal. If instruments are exchanged frequently the sheaths may be removed with the instrument. This results in a rapid loss of the

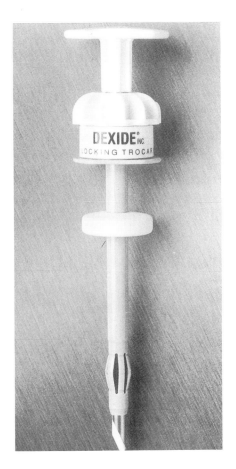

Fig. 3.14 Dexide self-stabilizing trocar.

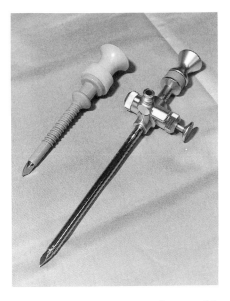

Fig. 3.15 A 5-mm trumpet valve reusable trocar and sheath (right) and a 5-mm simple disposable trocar (left).

pneumatoperitoneum and a significant delay whilst this is re-established and the trocar reinserted. Operating problems can also be encountered if the opposite occurs and the trocar sheath slips further into the cavity than intended. This may obstruct the proper opening of instruments and produce operating difficulties. Some of Ethicon's disposable trocar sheaths have a gripping device in the form of a screw thread on the outer surface of the cannula. USSC have a similar, separate, gripping device which can slide over their regular smooth cannula. These devices should ensure that the sheath remains in the correct position throughout the procedure. An alternative and ingenious atraumatic method of fixing the cannulae has been introduced by Dexide (Fig. 3.14). The trocar is inserted in the standard way and then a device on the collar of the cannula is rotated and a stabilizing collar protrudes to ensure that the device cannot then be inadvertently withdrawn from the abdomen. The device is prevented from slipping too far into the cavity by positioning a friction collar.

The insertion of the primary trocar is invariably a blind, and therefore potentially hazardous, procedure. In high-risk patients, a technique for direct or 'open' laparoscopy has been described by Harrith Hasson [1]. The technique of inserting this type of trocar is described in detail in Chapter 4. This type of instrument permits laparoscopy to be undertaken in relative safety in circumstances which might otherwise have represented a contraindication to laparoscopy.

Laparoscopic trocars usually have some form of valve mechanism to prevent excessive loss of gas. The most airtight but most inconvenient design is that of the trumpet valve (Fig. 3.15). With this design the trumpet valve must be depressed during insertion of any instrument. The firm grip of the valve also prevents the free movement of secondary instruments during surgery. We do not recommend this very common design of trocar for advanced laparoscopic procedures. Some form of flap valve, as used in the disposable trocar sheaths made by USSC and Ethicon, is much more convenient and appropriate for this form of surgery (Fig. 3.16). For secondary punctures with 5-mm instruments, we have found the shorter-length, screw-sheath, disposable trocars produced by Apple (Bolton, MA) very satisfactory and economical except when the patient is very obese (Fig. 3.17).

Recommendations

For the blind, primary, trocar insertion, a sharp 10-mm, flap-valved, disposable trocar with a protective sheath covering the tip and with a screw-fixing device on the sheath is to be preferred. For the secondary puncture sites, protective coverings for the tips are not required and a short-length trocar with simple flap valves and fixing device is recommended.

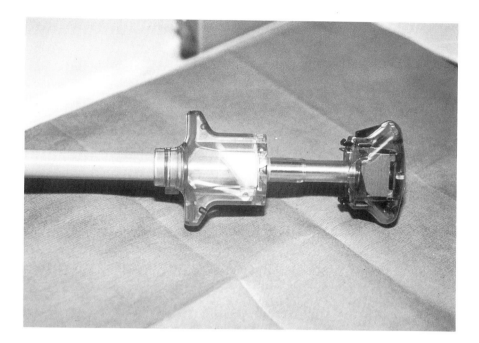

Fig. 3.16 An Ethicon 10-mm flap valve trocar sheath with demonstration transparent housing showing how the spring-loaded valve is pushed open by the trocar.

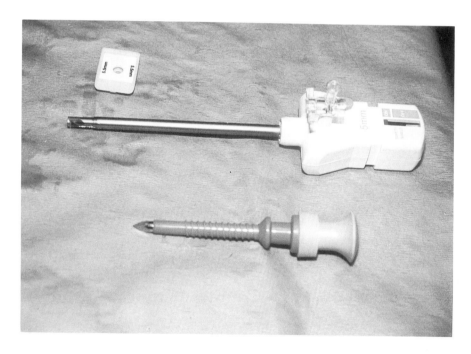

Fig. 3.17 An Apple 5-mm trocar (below) and 5-mm AutoSuture/USSC trocar (above).

Operative instruments

As the scope of laparoscopic procedures increases, so the range of equipment needed to perform these operations also increases. The manufacturers are responding to this challenge and at this present time there is an avalanche of new products coming on to the market which is threatening to engulf those who try to keep abreast with the latest developments.

Grasping forceps

It is just as essential in laparoscopic surgery as in open surgery to be able to gently and yet securely lift and manipulate tissues. A variety of different tissue-grasping forceps must be available in both 5- and 10-mm sizes. The smaller-diameter instruments are the basic work-horse instruments for advanced laparoscopic procedures and the 10-mm instruments are only used when large volumes of tissue must be grasped or removed.

Tissues which are not to be removed must be manoeuvred, displaced and held without damage. Various patterns of atraumatic grasping forceps are required. Semm has designed curved atraumatic forceps which are ideal for picking up the round ligament and the fallopian tube, and these are described in detail in the next chapter. Kleppinger-type forceps have been widely used in the US for electrosterilization and are also quite effective atraumatic graspers (Fig. 3.18). For thinner tissues, flat atraumatic forceps are useful (Fig. 3.19), and multiple-pronged, Hasson-type atraumatic graspers are especially useful for picking up the ovary (Fig. 3.20). The nose of the forceps may be sharp, round or flat, depending on the particular function (Fig. 3.21). It is useful to have some of these forceps with either a self-closing or a ratchet design so that they can be held closed on tissue for considerable periods of time without discomfort to the assistant (Fig. 3.22).

When a secure grasp is essential, toothed or rigid forceps are required. Semm has produced a toothed forceps which gives excellent grip by inserting a sharp pin, contained at the end of each jaw of the forceps, into the tissues (Fig. 3.23).

The large 10-mm claw forceps are useful for grasping and removing substantial portions of tissue through large trocars. This is particularly useful after morcellation of fibroids or solid ovarian tumours (Fig. 3.24).

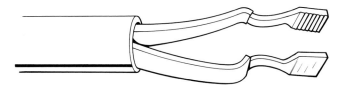

Fig. 3.18 Kleppinger bipolar forceps.

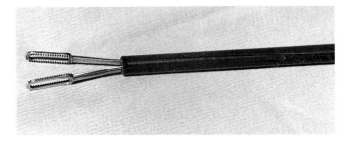

Fig. 3.19 Flat atraumatic forceps.

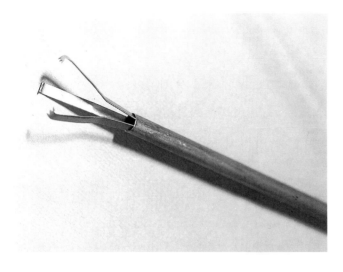

Fig. 3.20 Three-pronged Hassen grasping forceps.

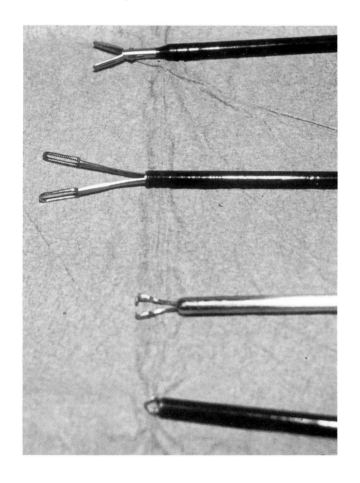

Fig. 3.21 Various shaped grasping forceps.

Curved dissecting forceps of various patterns are now available. We have found the 45° and 90° Petlin forceps (Wolfe, Germany) useful, particularly for skeletonizing vascular pedicles.

Needle-holders with appropriate ridges are essential for intra-abdominal suturing. Various conventional designs have been introduced

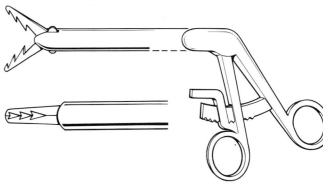

Fig. 3.22 Ratchet, self-retaining forceps.

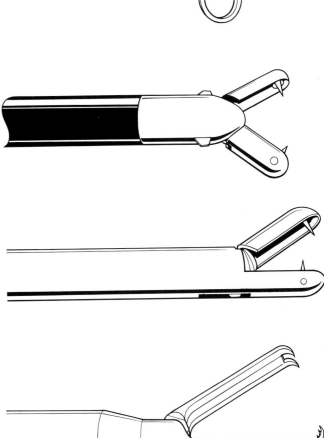

Fig. 3.23 Single-toothed grasping forceps.

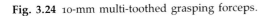

Fig. 3.24 10-mm multi-toothed grasping forceps.

on to the market recently and Cook (Cook Ob/Gyn, Spencer, IN) have produced a more unconventional set of three laparoscopic needle-drivers with firm, self-closing jaws, which provide for very secure laparoscopic suturing (Fig. 3.25).

Scissors

The standard scissors for laparoscopic surgery are the 5-mm hook scissors. These are used for most cutting of tissues such as adhesions, ovarian capsule or broad ligament and also for cutting ligatures. For

delicate dissection, microscissors are available. These are capable of
very fine work but should be used with caution because their points
are sharp and can easily damage bowel etc. during insertion. Flat
scissors are also useful for dividing tissues such as the peritoneum and
reflecting bladder flaps (Fig. 3.26). Laparoscopic scissors are usually of
single-action design and only one of the blades moves to perform
the cutting. Most surgeons are used to twin-action scissors with
both blades moving. USSC/AutoSuture have introduced a range of
laparoscopic shears which have fairly large twin-action blades. In common with other disposable products, they are also consistently sharp
and can be recommended in circumstances when this is important,
for it is notoriously difficult to keep stainless-steel reusable scissors
sharp.

Recommendation

A full range of grasping and dissecting forceps, needle-holders and
scissors are required before embarking upon laparoscopic surgery.

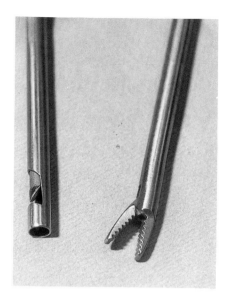

Fig. 3.25 Needle holders. Continental
toothed needle-holder (right) and a Cook
needle driver (left).

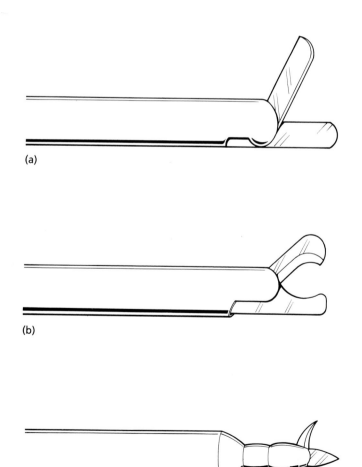

(a)

(b)

(c)

Fig. 3.26 (a) Straight scissors, (b) standard dissecting scissors
and (c) microscissors.

Clips and staples

A single or multiple clip applier may be an important emergency instrument because such systems can be the most rapid and effective method of occluding an isolated bleeding vessel. Such appliers place single 6-mm titanium clips on the structure to be occluded. The single applier can be a frustrating instrument to use for, although it is economical and reusable, it requires frequent removal for reloading, which can sometimes be difficult, particularly in the presence of active bleeding. Automatic multiclip appliers have now been produced by Ethicon and USSC (Fig. 3.27). These instruments contain 20 titanium clips and each can be loaded into the jaws without removing the instrument from the operative field, with significant savings both in operative time and surgeon's stress.

A disposable GIA stapling device (Endo GIA, USSC/AutoSuture, Norwalk, CT) is a most useful new endoscopic surgical device. The instrument fires two triple rows of staples and almost simultaneously divides the tissue between its jaws to produce haemostatic pedicles. The action of this device is fully described in the next chapter.

Morcellation

One of the major difficulties in laparoscopic surgery is to remove large volumes of tissue such as fibroids or ovarian tissue from the cavity after they have been excised. One way of doing this is to reduce the tissue into manageable portions. This can be done simply by cutting the tumour into pieces with scissors, laser or any other convenient

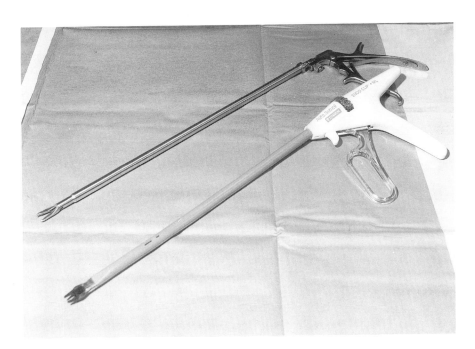

Fig. 3.27 Clip appliers. Single reusable clip applicator (top) and automatic, multiclip applicator (bottom).

modality. Kurt Semm has devised two types of morcellator to help with this problem. His first morcellator is made of two concentric hollow tubes, the inner of which contains a knife at its distal end (Fig. 3.28(a), (b)). When the handle of the device is pulled, the inner tube is drawn up into the outer tube. Tissue placed in the mouth of the morcellator will be cut and forced up the inner hollow tube (Fig. 3.29). Many passes will reduce the bulk of a tumour, which progressively becomes stored in the barrel of the morcellator. This tissue can subsequently be removed and sent for regular histological examination. Semm has more recently described a larger morcellator which he calls the serrated-edge macromorcellator (SEMM). This device is a large-diameter cylinder with a sharp, wave-shaped distal edge. A myoma screw or large claw-tooth forceps is inserted down the shaft and the tissue to be removed is pulled up whilst a cylinder is removed by forcing the serrated cutting edge of the morcellator into the tissue with a rotary movement. Other ways of reducing the volume of tissue are now being explored and among the most promising is a technique using ultrasound.

Recommendation

It is important to have one or more techniques to reduce tissue volume

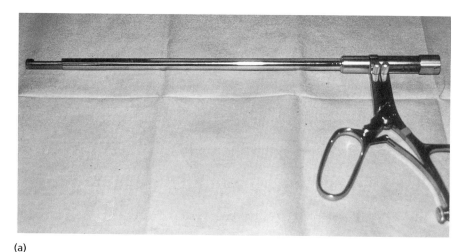

(a)

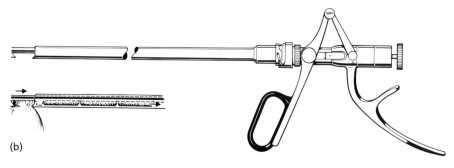

(b)

Fig. 3.28 (a) Semm morcellator. (b) Mode of action of Semm morcellator. Reproduced with permission from Sanfilippo JS, Levine RC (eds) *Operative Gynecologic Endoscopy*. Springer-Verlag, New York, 1989.

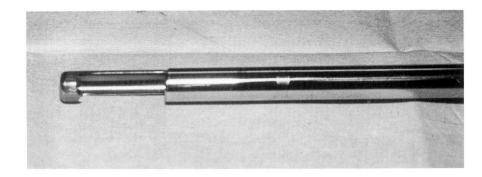

Fig. 3.29 Close up of Semm morcellator.

to facilitate extraction of large tissue specimens from the abdominal cavity through the standard laparoscopic incisions.

Suction irrigator—dissector

An efficient suction irrigator—dissector or aquadissector is one of the most important of all pieces of equipment for laparoscopic surgery. It is essential to maintain excellent vision in the presence of bleeding, and equipment capable of removing large volumes of fluid from the cavity quickly is mandatory. The aquadissector must also be able to rapidly force significant quantities of Ringer's lactate or normal saline into the abdomen to cleanse the site and flush away any blood, fluid, debris or smoke. This device can also be used as an excellent dissector and to hold and apply traction to tissues.

The simplest of such systems is to suspend the irrigating fluid bag from a pole and allow the fluid to flow into the cavity under gravity. In this system, flow rate can be regulated by altering the height of the bag. This infusion system can be improved by wrapping a blood-pressure cuff around the infusion bag. The more effective irrigators are powered by pressurized CO_2. This drives fluid from sterile reservoirs into the patient. The pressure can be varied and one of 300 mmHg is usually optimum. This allows a relatively rapid flow of fluid, capable of breaking up blood clots. The irrigation probes may have separate channels for suction and irrigation or may have a single channel to be used alternatively for both functions. The authors prefer the latter system as the channel is twice the diameter and therefore much faster and more efficient and capable of removing larger blood clots.

Recommendation

A CO_2-powered aquadissector with a large single probe is a most important piece of laparoscopic equipment.

Electrosurgery and lasers in endoscopic surgery

Many gynaecologists are apprehensive about using electrosurgical techniques laparoscopically again when they recall the severe complications which occurred when unipolar diathermy techniques were commonly used for fallopian-tube coagulation. Many gynaecologists are also apprehensive about using expensive laser equipment with which they are unfamiliar. Both modalities, however, have properties which make them very important and useful tools for use in advanced laparoscopic surgery.

Both electrosurgical and laser equipment consists of tools which can cut, coagulate and vaporize tissue. The fact that they are able to cut and coagulate almost simultaneously allows tissues to be divided without bleeding. Electrosurgery uses electrons to cut and coagulate whilst lasers use photons to achieve a similar effect. A scalpel cuts tissue by splitting it but lasers and electrosurgical devices both act like a saw and physically remove tissue to produce the cutting effect.

High-frequency electrosurgery

High-frequency (HF) electrical energy has been used for over 50 years to cut and coagulate biological tissues, using the intrinsic thermal effect of electrical current. To avoid inadvertent muscle and nerve stimulation, an alternating current of over 300 kHz must be used. Electrosurgical generators can produce current in three separate waveforms. The cutting waveform is an unmodulated sinus wave. Cutting will only occur when the voltage between the electrode and the tissue is high enough to produce an arc. Such an arc effectively concentrates the energy on to specific points of the tissue. The temperature at these points of contact is so high that the tissue is immediately vaporized. A voltage of more than 200 volts is required to produce such electric arcs and above this value arcs increase in proportion to the voltage. The greater the voltage, the deeper the depth of tissue coagulation.

Types of waveform

Cutting

To produce a cutting effect in biological tissues it is necessary to have a voltage sufficiently high to produce electric arcs between the cutting electrode and the tissue. The voltage is produced in an unmodulated (continuous) sinusoidal manner (Fig. 3.30(a)). The thickness and shape of the electrode also influences the type of tissue effect obtained and the most satisfactory cutting is produced with thin-edged needle or knife electrodes (Fig. 3.30(b)). This production of arcs generates points of extremely high local temperatures which result in immediate tissue

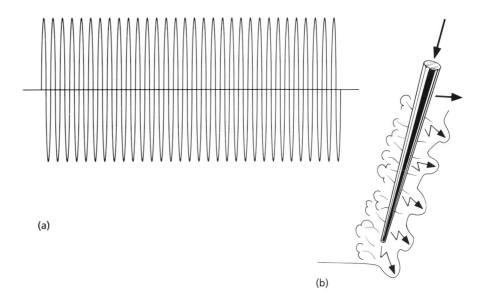

Fig. 3.30 (a) Continuous sinusoidal cutting current (low voltage, high frequency). (b) Arcs producing local tissue vaporization and cutting.

vaporization. Where the tissue is vaporized, a cutting effect is observed. Because the tissue is heated swiftly, there is insufficient time for heat to dissipate to adjacent tissue. This results in cutting without significant haemostasis.

Coagulation

Coagulation effects may be described as desiccation or fulguration, depending on the waveform, the manner in which it is applied and the shape of the electrode. Coagulation is produced with higher voltages than used for cutting but the flow is applied intermittently with it switched off or modulated for a proportion of the time. This modulation or damping effectively slows the heating of the tissues by allowing the tissues to cool between bursts of heating (Fig. 3.31). This reduces the net local heating effect to below that required to produce tissue vaporization. The higher the voltage used and the longer the modulation intervals, the greater the coagulation effect and consequently the greater the haemostatic effect.

Blended waveform is a combination of cutting and coagulation

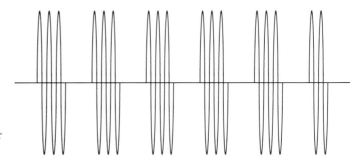

Fig. 3.31 Modulated coagulation current (higher voltage, lower frequency).

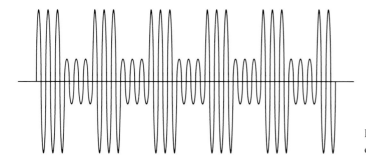

Fig. 3.32 Blended waveform with a combination of cutting and coagulation waveforms.

forms. It consists of bursts of alternating high and low voltage and produces a cutting effect with some coagulation (Fig. 3.32).

Desiccation. Tissues are coagulated when they are heated to between 70 and 100°C and this process is called desiccation. Soft coagulation is characterized by the fact that no electric arcs are produced between the electrode and the tissue. Unmodulated (cutting) voltages below the trigger value for arcing (200 V) should be used to produce this effect. Soft coagulation should be used whenever an electrode is brought into direct contact with the tissue to be coagulated. Soft coagulation may be produced with either unipolar or bipolar electrodes. Unipolar coagulation can be produced with ball- or spatula-shaped electrodes or with grasping forceps applied to the tissues. Bipolar coagulation can only be applied between two blades of a pair of forceps. To coagulate large blood-vessels it is important to continue the flow of current until the tissues are completely desiccated and current can no longer flow. It is, however, equally important to stop the desiccation at this time, to avoid the coagulum adhering to the electrode and subsequently being torn from the vessels, with consequent inadequate haemostasis. This optimum coagulation is best achieved either by monitoring the flow of current or by using an automatic cut and coagulation surgical unit (to be described in a subsequent chapter).

Fulguration. Forced coagulation occurs when electric arcs are deliberately produced between the electrode and the tissue. This process is called fulguration and is produced when a coagulation current is applied in the non-contact mode with a space between the active electrode and the tissue. The current follows a path of least resistance and arcs to the tissue to produce a deeper coagulation than that associated with soft coagulation. The depth of the coagulation is proportional to the length of the arcs, which in turn is proportional to the voltage used. This type of coagulation is also associated with greater char formation and should only be used in specific circumstances.

Spray coagulation is the extreme form of fulguration and occurs when long electric arcs are deliberately produced. Strongly modulated HF voltages with high voltage levels are required to produce this type of effect. Spray coagulation can be used to produce a relatively superficial coagulation.

Early electrosurgical generators that produced this type of tissue effect contained two separate generators. A vacuum-tube generator produced unmodulated HF voltage for cutting with little coagulation and a spark-gap generator produced strongly amplitude-modulated HF voltage for cutting with intensive coagulation. Recently constructed generators are controlled by semiconductors. These do not need to mix the outputs of two separate generators but simply control with microprocessors the amplitude and degree of modulation of the current generated.

Modern generators which produce cutting and coagulation currents efficiently and effectively include Valleylab SSE2L (Valleylab, Boulder, CO) and Aspen Excalibur (Aspen Labs, Englewood, CO). A new type of electrosurgical generator which may be of particular value in advanced endoscopic surgery is the Erbotom ACC 454 (Erbe Elektromedizin GmbH, Tübingen, Germany). This machine measures the intensity of the electrical arcs with microprocessor technology and adjusts the output to produce the desired cutting and coagulation effect automatically. These newer machines can monitor and warn of any potentially dangerous low-frequency leaks of current from the patient to earth and any high-frequency leaks of current, for example via metal stands or operating-room (OR) table poles to earth. Such leakages can cause excess local heating and severe burns. Modern generators can also, by means of split-return electrodes, warn of incomplete application of the return electrode. These warning devices significantly reduce but do not abolish the risks of using high-frequency currents.

Argon-beam coagulator. A conventional spray coagulation current can arc for 1–2 mm. If the point electrode is placed in a stream of inert argon gas, the electrons will be carried on the argon stream and can produce a coagulation arc for up to 10 mm (Fig. 3.33). The argon beam coagulator uses this principle and can be used laparoscopically (Fig. 3.34). An advantage of this system is that the flow of argon gas flushes away surface blood and debris and makes visualization of the bleeding point more precise. The jet of argon is a coolant and there is correspondingly less smoke generated than with standard electrosurgery. The flow of argon must be controlled and the abdominal cavity frequently vented to reduce the risks of an air embolism. The risk of this complication has not yet been established and the role of this technique in laparoscopic surgery is not yet certain.

Recommendation

There have been major advances in electrosurgical equipment in the last few years. The Erbotom ACC 450 automatic cut-and-coagulation

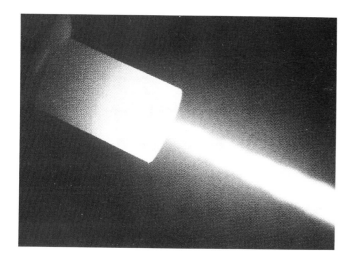

Fig. 3.33 Stream of argon gas carrying electrons to tissue to produce superficial coagulation.

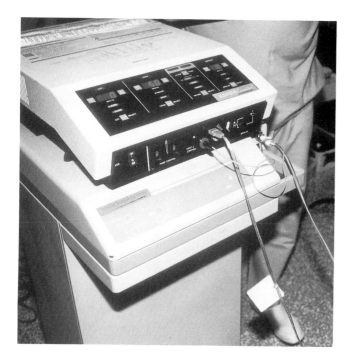

Fig. 3.34 An argon beam coagulator with associated Aspen electrosurgical generator.

unit represents the state-of-the-art system which presents some exciting opportunities.

Lasers in advanced endoscopic surgery

To some, lasers remain overpriced technology which can do nothing that cannot be achieved with simpler, less expensive equipment. To others, however, lasers have properties which are clinically valuable and many feel they have a place in the armamentarium of an endoscopic surgeon. Professor Bruhat from Clermont-Ferrand in France first introduced the CO_2 laser into laparoscopic surgery [2]. He believes that the two technologies of laparoscopy and lasers represent two efficient, elegant and atraumatic techniques which can provide considerable practical and economic benefits to the patients. Lasers are, however, costly pieces of equipment and can perhaps only be justified in larger units with high patient through-puts. In these circumstances, the cost of the laser expressed in terms of the cost per case may be acceptably and sometimes surprisingly low.

The laser uses photons to dissect and coagulate tissue. In general, lasers produce less lateral tissue damage than that produced by electrosurgery. Lasers used in laparoscopic surgery are either solid-state or gas lasers. The gas lasers with gaseous active medium include the CO_2 and argon ion (Ar^+) lasers. The solid-state lasers have a solid active medium and include the neodymium-doped yttrium−aluminium−garnet (Nd-YAG) laser. Laserscope (Laserscope, San Jose, CA) have directed an Nd-YAG laser through a crystal of potassium-titanyl-phosphate (KTP). This crystal doubles the frequency of the Nd-YAG laser and produces a beam with a wavelength which is half that of the original.

All lasers produce monochromatic light but this fact is less important than the position of the laser wavelength in the electromagnetic spectrum. All lasers also produce coherent light, with all the waves in phase. This coherence is not, however, of importance to the surgeon, for coherence is usually lost during passage down a fibreoptic or between mirrors.

Carbon dioxide lasers

The first laser to be used in gynaecological endoscopy was the CO_2 laser. This was used more or less independently by Bruhat in France [2], Tadir in Israel [3], Daniell and Brown in the US [4], and Sutton in the UK [5]. The CO_2 laser, with a wavelength of 10 600 nm, is in the far-infrared portion of the electromagnetic spectrum. It can only be transmitted from the laser generator to the endoscope by a system of articulated arms containing six or seven metallic mirrors. These mirrors should be precisely aligned to preserve the configuration and the power of the beam. At the distal end of the articulated arm, the beam must be delivered into the abdomen. This may be connected either directly to the operating channel of the laparoscope or down a secondary channel. The advantage of the single-puncture approach is that the path of the laser beam closely parallels the operator's line of vision, facilitating precise aiming of the beam. The disadvantage of this system is that some of the optical channel must be given up to accommodate the operating channel, with a corresponding reduction in image brightness. The double-puncture approach conversely maximizes visual conditions but at the cost of demanding greater operator skill to aim the beam.

Previously the beam was coupled to the laparoscope or secondary trocar sheath via a pivoted-mirror type of joy-stick micromanipulator. This system was difficult to align and the beam frequently struck the sides of the sheath with consequent loss of power. To overcome this difficulty with the second-puncture approach, Sutton suggested the use of shortened probes with a fixing device, making a micromanipulator unnecessary [5]. The focal length of the system is set to focus the beam 10 mm beyond the distal end of the probe. Infraguide quartz fibres (LaserSonics, Santa Clara, CA) have been introduced so that the CO_2 beam can be transmitted down this semiflexible fibre. It is claimed that 90% of the CO_2 energy can be transmitted down the waveguide but unfortunately CO_2 is invisible and an aiming beam is also required. Less than 50% of the usual He−Ne aiming beam is transmitted down such a guide and this makes accurate use of this laser difficult. This particular problem now appears to have been overcome by the development of new coupling devices. These devices are constructed to ensure that the laser beam is maintained directly down the centre of the operating channel and the beam can therefore be maintained in perfect alignment (see Fig. 3.10).

Smoke and plume can accumulate in the operating channel of the scope but this can be cleared by purging the channel with a continuous flow of CO_2 gas. The purging gas itself decreases the power of the CO_2 laser beam delivered to the tissue because the wavelength of the purging gas is the same as that of the laser. This has been shown to reduce the power delivered by 30−60%. The passage also increases the effective size of the laser spot and this 'blooming' effect further reduces the power effect at the tissue. Coherent have recently overcome this problem by altering the wavelength of the CO_2 laser, through the use of an isotope of CO_2, from 10.6 µm to 11.1 µm (Ultrapulse 5000L). This subtle change in wavelength means that the purge gas no longer interferes with the laser power and that the blooming effect is much reduced.

Unwanted damage to tissues lateral to the site of beam impact is produced by heat conduction and is related to the time of exposure to the thermal insult. The longer the exposure, the more tissue damage and charring which will occur. To minimize the duration of exposure, the superpulse mode was developed. With superpulse, very high-power (500 W), low-energy pulses are released for brief surges (2 mJ), with longer intervals between to allow the tissues to cool. Ultrapulse is a similar system which delivers very high-energy pulses (200 mJ) at the same high power levels as superpulse (500 W) to allow even longer cooling intervals between pulses.

The main endoscopic uses for the CO_2 laser are based on the ability of a CO_2 beam to cut very precisely with minimal lateral tissue damage. This is of great value in, for example, dissection on the pelvic side-wall near the ureter and for precise incisions around the fallopian tubes in infertility surgery. The vaporization capability of the laser can be used to remove implants of endometriosis.

Recommendation

A high-power superpulse or ultrapulse CO_2 laser with a reliable coupling device is recommended. The Coherent 5000L has been specifically designed for laparoscopic surgery and appears to be the state-of-the-art device at the time of writing.

Fibre lasers

The articulated arms used for CO_2 lasers are bulky and subject to mechanical misalignments. Many surgeons prefer a flexible, fibre, delivery system as it is simpler to use, cannot become misaligned and can readily reach remote tissues. Light from a fibreoptic diverges as it moves away from the fibre tip. The angle of divergence is about $15°$, which means the spot size will grow about 1 mm for every 4 mm distance the fibre is moved from the tissue. Nd-YAG, KTP and argon lasers can all be transmitted down quartz fibres.

Nd-YAG laser

The Nd-YAG laser has a wavelength of 1.06 μm, which is in the near-infrared (and invisible) portion of the electromagnetic spectrum. When transmitted down a bare quartz fibre, the Nd-YAG laser energy penetrates deeply into tissue. This property may be of considerable value in certain circumstances, such as in ablating the endometrium for the treatment of dysfunctional uterine bleeding. It may, however, be of considerable inconvenience or even danger when used inside the abdominal cavity. Joffe designed a series of artificial ceramic 'sapphire' tips and these are marketed by Surgical Laser Technology (Malvern, PA). These tips essentially focus the laser beam so that tissue penetration and scatter are markedly reduced. The envelope of energy distribution is dependent on the shape of the tip and various shapes can be used to tailor the tip to the indication (Fig. 3.35). This system, with the tips mounted on long, semirigid handpieces, restores to the laser surgeon the sensation of touch. Smoke production is very much less with this modality than with the CO_2 laser or electrosurgery, and the Nd-YAG laser produces a much greater coagulation effect on small blood-vessels than that achieved with the CO_2 laser. With scalpel-shaped tips, the amount of unintended tissue damage of 0.2−1.0 mm is similar to that achieved with the 'what you see is what you get' type of tissue destruction associated with the use of the CO_2 laser.

These sapphire probes and handpieces are highly engineered and correspondingly expensive. They must withstand tremendous tempera-

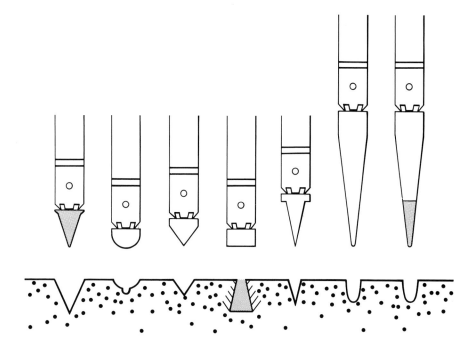

Fig. 3.35 The effect on tissue of different shaped sapphire tips.

tures and need to be cooled. The handpieces have coaxial conduits for gas or liquid cooling. CO_2 gas is the most convenient agent for cooling but must be used with care. Excessive flow will raise the pressure in the abdominal cavity, with the risk of air embolism and subcutaneous emphysema.

If the invisible Nd-YAG laser beam is inadvertently directed into the eye, the wavelength will pass through the cornea and anterior chamber of the eye to be focused on to the retina, with disastrous consequences. To prevent this, protective goggles should be worn. These are usually of a green colour, with an optical density of at least 5, but more expensive, almost clear goggles are a preferred option.

Recommendation

The Nd-YAG laser can be used laparoscopically to provide good cutting with simultaneous haemostasis and can also be used to vaporize tissue. This wavelength should only be used with a focusing system, and currently the best such system appears to be the sapphire tips manufactured by Surgical Laser Technology.

KTP laser

The potassium-titanyl-phosphate (KTP) laser produces a visible beam in the blue-green portion of the visible spectrum at a wavelength of 532 nm. This wavelength passes down a flexible fibre, passes through clear fluids and penetrates tissues for about 1–2 mm. This is greater tissue penetration than occurs with CO_2 or with Nd-YAG used with sapphire tips but less than with Nd-YAG with a bare fibre. The KTP laser produces cutting with good simultaneous haemostasis, with minimal associated smoke production and without the need for expensive tips. It does not vaporize or cut tissue as fast as the CO_2 laser or coagulate as well as the Nd-YAG laser, but the KTP modality can perform all three functions with a single, bare, quartz fibre which can be used repeatedly.

The protective goggles required for this laser are a distracting pink colour. Also it is essential to insert a protective filter in the optic pathway to protect the video system and this reduces the available light. The KTP laser needs three-phase electricity and some earlier models also required running water as a coolant. The principal disadvantage of this system, however, is its high initial cost, as the KTP laser is the most expensive of the commonly used machines.

Argon laser

The argon laser was the first laser to be used in medicine. In 1964 it was used in the eye to treat intraocular haemorrhages and detached retinae. The visible blue-green beam, at 488 nm, passes down a flexible quartz fibre and can easily be led into the abdominal cavity. The argon laser is a gas discharge which requires extremely high electrical current densities, in excess of 100 A/cm, passing through the gas to excite the laser discharge. In spite of this, the argon laser is less powerful than the others discussed here and it must be water-cooled, which is a major inconvenience.

Recommendation

These KTP and argon lasers are at wavelengths in the same portion of the visible blue-green area of the electromagnetic spectrum. They have many similar properties and clinical effects, but the KTP is more powerful and flexible because it can also produce a bare-fibre, Nd-YAG laser effect.

Ultrasonic cutting and coagulation system

One of the most recent modalities developed which may have a function in laparoscopic surgery is the introduction by UltraCision Inc. (Smithfield, RI) of an ultrasonically activated scalpel, which has recently been adapted for laparoscopic use. It is claimed that this device also permits simultaneous cutting and coagulation. The disposable blade of the Harmonic scalpel moves rapidly back and forth, producing an almost imperceptible sawing motion 55 000 times per second. This mechanical motion causes the collagen molecules to vibrate and become a coagulum. This tissue coagulum occurs with minimal heat because it is generated directly in the tissue and not at the blade. The blade remains cool and the tissue temperature near the blade rises to 80–90°C. This results in minimal tissue damage and no charring or smoke production. Small blood-vessels are sealed by the direct action of the blade. Larger vessels up to 3 mm in diameter can be occluded by pressing the side of the blade on to the vessel, thereby tamponading it. The subsequent application of a short burst of high-power ultrasonic vibration seals it.

Recommendation

This is interesting but as yet unproved technology.

Summary

A great many pieces of equipment have been described in this chapter. All are interesting, many will be helpful but not all are essential. What is essential is that the surgeon has access to excellent visualization equipment and to an automatic, high-flow, pneumatoperitoneal insufflation apparatus. Several different methods of tissue division and haemostasis must also be available and a reliable suction–irrigation device is indispensable. Laparoscopic atraumatic and sharp graspers, scissors and suturing equipment are also essential. Many of the more advanced procedures will be difficult without either an adequate laparoscopic diathermy or an efficient laser system, and ideally both modalities should be immediately at hand.

It is clear that these procedures cannot be attempted just with the equipment most gynaecologists are familiar with and use for diagnostic laparoscopy. Advanced laparoscopic techniques can offer major benefits to the patients and considerable financial savings can also be made. However, these benefits cannot be obtained on the cheap and considerable capital outlay is required before such procedures can safely be attempted. The whole minimally invasive laparoscopic approach will rapidly become discredited if attempted using inadequate instrumentation. Clearly, education and training in these new techniques are also essential for a successful outcome, but this matter will be discussed in detail in a later chapter.

References

1 Hasson HM. Open laparoscopy. In: Sanfilippo JS, Levine RC (eds) *Operative Gynecologic Endoscopy*, pp. 57–67. Springer Verlag, New York, 1989.
2 Bruhat MA, Mage G, Manhes H. Use of the CO_2 laser by laparoscopy. In: Kaplan I (ed.) *Laser Surgery III*. Proceedings of the Third International Congress on Laser Surgery, pp. 275–281. Jerusalem Press, Tel Aviv, 1979.

3 Tadir Y, Kaplan I, Zuckerman K. A second puncture probe for laser laparoscopy. In: Atsumi K, Nimsakul N (eds) *Laser Surgery IV*. Proceedings of the Fourth Congress of the International Society for Laser Surgery, pp. 25–26. Japanese Society for Laser Medicine, Tokyo, 1981.

4 Daniell JF, Brown DH. Carbon dioxide laser laparoscopy: initial experience in experimental animals and humans. *Obstet Gynaecol* 1982; **59**: 761.

5 Sutton CJG. Initial experience with carbon dioxide laser laparoscopy. *Laser Med Sci* 1985; **1**: 25–31.

4: Basic Techniques for Advanced Laparoscopic Surgery

This chapter deals with many of the practical steps that are necessary for effective advanced laparoscopic surgery.

Preoperative preparation

Most laparoscopic procedures are performed on a day-case or short-stay basis. Rapid through-put of patients puts new demands on nursing and ancillary staff, as detailed in Chapter 13.

Patients who are to have surgery in the morning are requested to have nothing to eat or drink from 10.00 p.m. on the evening prior to surgery. Those for afternoon surgery are permitted a light breakfast. One of the authors feels it is important to ensure that the stomach is completely deflated by passing an orogastric tube prior to surgery. If extensive bowel dissection is anticipated, as for example in cases of stage 4 cul-de-sac endometriosis or if there is a history of major intra-abdominal adhesions, preoperative bowel preparation is also given. Routine shaving of pubic hair is not performed. If clinical examination has suggested a pelvic mass, pelvic or vaginal ultrasound examinations should be performed. Patients are encouraged to void immediately prior to surgery. A full pelvic examination is performed under anaesthesia to determine the size, position and mobility of the uterus and to exclude any ovarian or adnexal masses.

Positioning of the patient

Many operative laparoscopic procedures take a considerable time to complete. To avoid the risk of damage to the patient, to ensure the comfort of the operating team and to facilitate the procedure, the patient must be carefully and correctly positioned on the table. The buttocks must be placed on the edge of the table. This will allow for the greatest range of movement of the instruments placed inside the uterus for manipulation. The cervix may be grasped with a vulsellum forceps and a Spackman cannula inserted into the cavity and the two secured together. A better way to control uterine position is to insert a Valtchev uterine mobilizer (Figs 4.1 and 4.2) (Conkin Surgical, Toronto, Ont.). This instrument can rotate the uterus through the widest possible arc and also clearly delineate the posterior vaginal fornix, which is essential during some difficult cases.

The patient's legs must be abducted as fully as possible in order to maximize the space available between the legs. They are maintained in

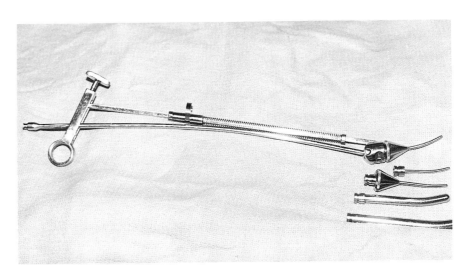

Fig. 4.1 Valtchev uterine mobilizer.

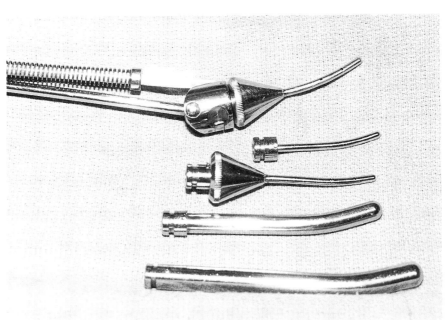

Fig. 4.2 Close up of interchangeable tips of a Valtchev uterine manipulator.

a low lithotomy position to allow the surgeon the maximum room at the patient's side and reduce the need for the surgeon to adopt an uncomfortable position. The arms should not be placed on an arm board but can be placed down the patient's side or folded across her chest. The steepest possible Trendelenberg position may be required to displace contents out of the pelvis. A manual tilt table capable of producing 30° of Trendelenberg is to be preferred. If such a position is to be maintained, supportive shoulder braces may also be required.

Recommendation

Care must be taken that the patient is positioned in a safe position which also permits the maximum comfortable access.

Establishment of the pneumatoperitoneum

A sharp Veress needle is inserted into the abdominal cavity (Fig. 4.3). The skin should be incised prior to this and the primary incision should be inside the umbilicus. If for some reason this site is unsuitable, the Veress needle may be inserted through the posterior fornix, although indications for this route are very few. A third route recommended by Reich in cases in which many lower abdominal adhesions may be anticipated is through the ninth left intercostal space. In such cases a pneumatoperitoneum is induced through this transthoracic route and a 5-mm diagnostic telescope can be inserted in the same site and the lower adhesions taken down before the usual telescope is inserted into the regular umbilical position.

Initial umbilical incision

Dr Hasson described the detailed surgical anatomy of the periumbilical abdominal wall [1]. He noted that, because of the unique events occurring in this area at the time of birth, the anatomy of this part of the abdominal wall is also unique. In this area there is no subcutaneous fat between the skin and deep fascia and these two layers are fused at this site. He suggests that the postnatal umbilical scar is drawn firmly against the umbilical ring and linea alba by fibrous cords representing redundant umbilical vessels and the urachus. During adult life the puckered skin of the umbilicus is retracted beneath the level of the skin of the rest of the abdominal wall. A retracted area within the lower border of the umbilicus represents the position where the skin is

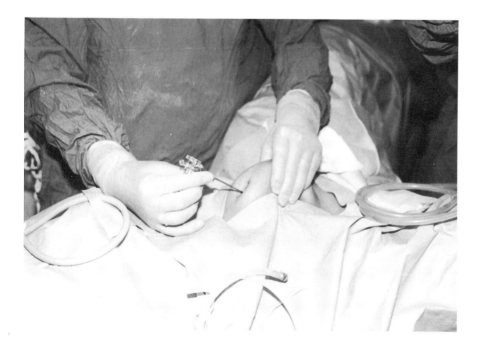

Fig. 4.3 Insertion of Veress needle through umbilical incision into the uterus.

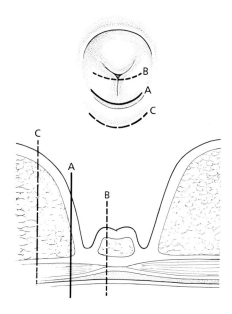

Fig. 4.4 Position of umbilical incision (after Hasson, 1989).

fused with the linea alba (Fig. 4.4). Incising the skin that overlies the lower margin of the umbilicus immediately exposes the linea alba portion of the deep fascia. Superiorly the fascia is fused with the skin but caudally the fascia is attached to the skin only with loose connective-tissue fibres. This natural cleavage plane defines a convenient site for laparoscopy.

In 1862 Langer described natural skin cleavage lines resulting from the natural disposition and alignment of collagen bundles in the skin. It is accepted that incisions made parallel to these lines heal better and gape less than incisions that cut across these lines. Langer's lines spread out in a sunburst formation from the umbilicus. Two studies have shown that vertical incisions heal better than transverse ones. In thin patients the initial incision may also cut through the deep fascia but the risk of intraperitoneal injury at this time can be reduced by rolling the umbilicus on to the surgeon's forefinger to control the depth of the incision.

Recommendation

The first incision for the primary trocar should be a vertical one, commencing in the umbilical fossa and extending caudally for 10 mm.

Inserting the Veress needle

After cleansing the abdomen, vulva and vagina with suitable antiseptic skin preparation, the Veress needle is connected to the CO_2 insufflator and tested for patency by observing a free flow of gas. A right-handed surgeon will then pick up the abdominal wall with his left hand and raise it away from the abdominal contents. The insertion is through the thinnest portion of the abdominal wall where the peritoneum is firmly attached to the underlying fascia, making it less likely to 'peel off' and produce an extraperitoneal infusion of gas. Experienced laparoscopists can usually feel the needle make a 'double pop' as it passes through the fascia and the peritoneum to enter the peritoneal cavity. If the needle is free in the cavity, it can readily be moved around without resistance.

Checking the placement of the insufflation needle

Several tests have been described to determine if the needle is correctly sited and, if there is clinical doubt about this, one or more of the tests should be performed before proceeding with the insufflation:

1 *Hiss test*. This is the sound of air being drawn into the peritoneal cavity through the Veress needle as the anterior abdominal wall is elevated. Quite a rare thing in a modern operating theatre is the silence required to recognize this sign.

2 *Aspiration test.* A syringe filled with normal saline is connected to the Veress needle. Fluid injected into the abdominal cavity cannot be aspirated back unless the needle remains in the abdominal wall. Pure blood or bowel contents will obviously indicate an incorrect siting of the needle.

3 *Sniff test.* If the bowel has been penetrated, foul-smelling gas may be detected; this should be detected before insufflation begins.

4 *Early insufflation pressure test.* If the gas is flowing freely, the rate of flow on the dial should correspond to that anticipated and the intra-abdominal pressure recorded should not exceed 8 mmHg at an infusion rate of 1 litre/min. Rising pressures and pressures above 15 mmHg associated with little or no flow indicate an incorrectly positioned needle.

5 *Palmer's test.* After induction of the pneumatoperitoneum, a needle connected to a glass syringe half-filled with normal saline is inserted into the cavity (Fig. 4.5). If bubbles of gas cannot be withdrawn, it is likely that adhesions or omentum are surrounding the entry point and insertion of the trocar at that point should be avoided.

Recommendation

The Veress needle must be inserted with care and its correct positioning checked prior to the production of the pneumatoperitoneum.

Instillation of the pneumatoperitoneum

The infusion of CO_2 should begin at a rate of 1 litre/min until it is clear that there is no obstruction to its inflow and no rise in instillation

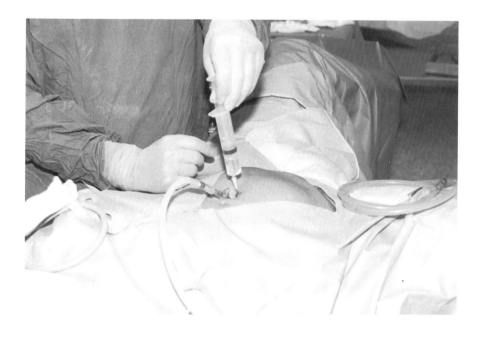

Fig. 4.5 Palmer's test. Withdrawing bubbles of CO_2 confirms needle is in free space in abdominal cavity.

pressure. When satisfactory placement is confirmed, faster flow can be produced. The rate of abdominal distension is usually limited by the diameter of the gas channel in the Veress needle rather than the rate of flow pumped out by the insufflator. Few Veress needles can permit abdominal distension at a rate in excess of 3 litres/min. During insufflation, the rate of flow, the pressure in the cavity and the volume of gas instilled are all monitored.

The gas flow is discontinued when:

1   the tension in the abdominal wall is judged to be adequate;
2   a standard volume of gas has been instilled;
3   a predetermined pressure has been achieved.

In a woman of average build, 3 litres of gas is usually sufficient to adequately distend the cavity. Once the required degree of distension is achieved, the maximum permitted abdominal pressure should be set and the insufflator set to the automatic mode. With this setting, gas is only instilled to replace that which is lost, and the degree of abdominal distension and the level of intrauterine pressure are maintained at constant preset levels. The optimum abdominal pressure during laparoscopic surgery varies according to patient build etc. but is usually between 12 and 15 mmHg.

Recommendation

CO_2 should be infused with care. The rate of gas flow and the intra-abdominal pressure should be continuously monitored and the latter should be maintained at a predetermined level of around 12 mmHg.

Insertion of the primary trocar

Inadvertent traumatic perforation of the bowel or a large vessel during the initial placement of the primary trocar is an inevitable risk of laparoscopic surgery. This risk may be minimized by good technique and the appropriate choice of instruments. In most instances the primary trocar will be 10 mm in diameter. It is essential that this trocar is sharp, and a pyramidal-shaped point will probably penetrate the abdominal wall more easily and therefore with more control than a blunt or conical-shaped point. It is at this moment of blind insertion that inadvertent damage to the bowel or major blood-vessels is most likely to occur. It is therefore at this moment that the spring-loaded shields which protect the trocar point after insertion through the abdominal wall may be of most value. If money for disposable items such as trocars is limited, it is suggested that the maximum benefit from the sharp, protected, disposable trocars produced by Ethicon and USSC/AutoSuture will be obtained from restricting their use to this primary trocar insertion (Fig. 4.6). Reich believes that deliberately increasing the intra-abdominal pressure to 25 mmHg at this time will thin the

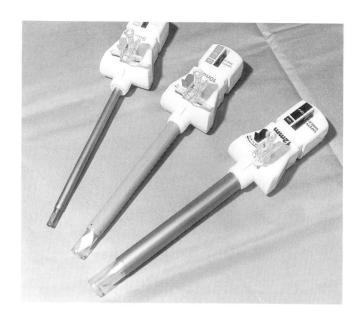

Fig. 4.6 A series of protected disposable trocars and sheaths recommended for primary insertion site.

abdominal wall and increase its tension, making the insertion of the trocar easier and more controlled and hence safer. If this technique is adopted, it is important to reduce the pressure to the standard 12–15 mmHg as soon as trocar insertion has been completed.

Once the appropriate trocar has been selected, it is grasped prior to insertion. The surgeon should place the handle of the trocar in his palm and then extend his index finger down the barrel of the trocar sheath so that only a small amount of the tip protrudes below (Fig. 4.7). With this grip the depth of possible penetration should be restricted to a safe amount. The trocar should be inserted at right angles to the skin

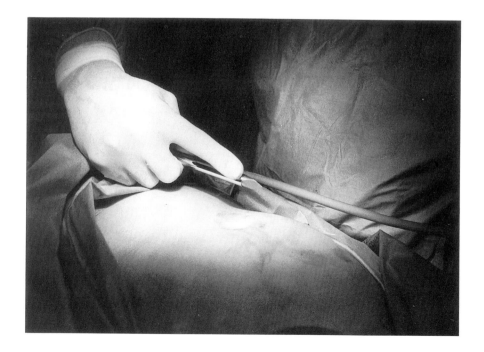

Fig. 4.7 Grip of trocar to prevent inadvertent insertion to too great depth.

(Fig. 4.8) and pushed vertically through the abdominal wall until the point just enters the cavity, when the direction of thrust should be changed to a horizontal direction (Fig. 4.9). This approach results in the parietal peritoneum being punctured directly beneath the umbilicus, so greatly reducing the amount of abdominal wall traversed. If the surgeon's hands are not big enough to adequately protect the trocar point, a different technique should be adopted. The trocar should enter the umbilical port and be directed down towards the pelvis at an angle

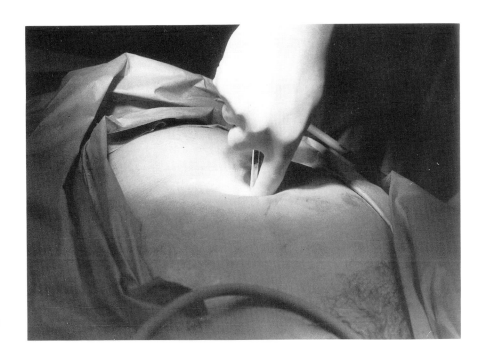

Fig. 4.8 Insertion of primary trocar at right angles to the abdominal skin in the umbilicus.

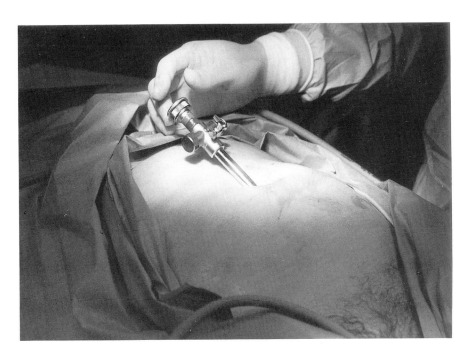

Fig. 4.9 Trocar insertion second stage — horizontal thrust.

of 45° and aiming at the position of the uterine fundus (Fig. 4.10). Approximately midway along this oblique track the trocar should be directed back towards the umbilicus so that the exit point emerges immediately below the entry.

For patients at risk of severe abdominal adhesions, Semm has described a technique of 'visually controlled peritoneal perforation' [2]. With this technique a 5-mm trocar with an oblique distal end is inserted carefully down to, but not through, the muscle layer of the abdominal wall. The trocar is then replaced with a 5-mm telescope and the trocar sheath advanced under visual control through the remainder of the muscle layer and down to the peritoneum. When the cavity beneath the peritoneum is clear of underlying problems, the peritoneum will be translucent. When bowel or omentum is adherent under the telescope, a dull white reflection will be seen. The trocar can then be manoeuvred until a safe translucent area is found. This translucent area can be punctured under direct vision with the sheath of the trocar.

A further alternative approach to initial trocar insertion in difficult cases is Hasson's 'open laparoscopy' [1]. He has developed an open-laparoscopy cannula which has a cone-shaped sleeve that slides freely over the cannula shaft. This cone can be fixed in any position on the shaft by tightening a screw. The distal end of the trocar obturator is rounded and blunt. The trocar cannula also has two V-shaped suture holders to permit anchorage of the cannula to the skin (Fig. 4.11). The device is inserted into a skin incision about 10 mm long. Using skin hooks and fine retractors to maintain vision, the incision is deepened by opening closed scissors until the fascia is seen. The fascia is elevated with a skin hook and then grasped with a Kocher's forceps and incised transversely. A strong suture is inserted into the fascia on each side. The peritoneal cavity is then entered, the cannula inserted and the cone secured at an appropriate position on the shaft. The sutures through the fascia are pulled upwards and threaded into the V-shaped suture holders of the cannula. This manoeuvre anchors the cannula firmly against the cone to provide an airtight seal. The gas line is connected and the blunt obturator withdrawn and replaced by a 10-mm telescope.

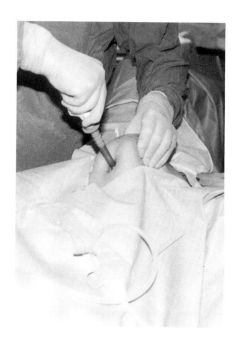

Fig. 4.10 Alternative primary trocar insertion for surgeons with small hands.

Recommendation

Insertion of the primary trocar is a blind procedure and is associated with a significant risk of bowel and blood-vessel injury. These risks can be minimized, but not abolished, by careful technique.

Secondary trocar sites

Between one and three lower abdominal sites are selected, depending on the procedure and technique employed. The two constant positions

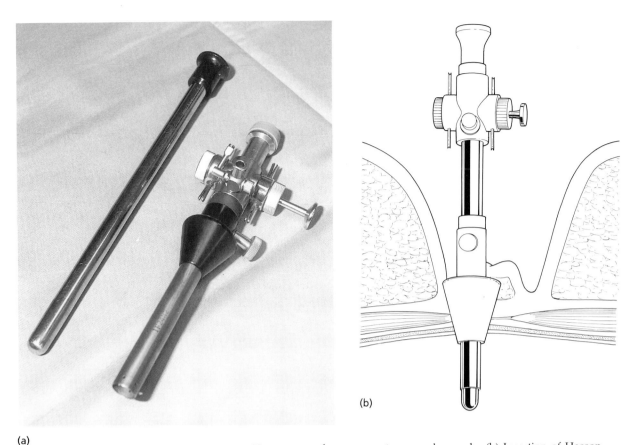

(a)

(b)

Fig. 4.11 (a) Hasson open laparoscope trocar and cannula. (b) Insertion of Hasson cannula. Reproduced with permission from Sanfilippo JS, Levine RC (eds). *Operative Gynecologic Endoscopy.* Springer-Verlag, New York, 1989.

employed for most advanced pelvic endoscopic surgery are in the right and left iliac fossae. If a third site is used, it will be located in the midline suprapubically. The left lower trocar site is the major portal for operative manipulation. The right lower trocar site is used mainly for retraction. The central portal is used either for accessory instruments or for the application of Endo GIA staples, when it will need to be 12 mm in length.

The position of the lateral lower portal sites should vary according to the size of the uterus and the procedure to be performed. For a normal-size uterus the incisions are placed two finger-breadths above the symphysis pubica. If the uterus is grossly enlarged or other pelvic pathology is anticipated, the level and position of the trocars may be varied to optimize the angle of approach. Such flexibility based on individual clinical features follows exactly the same principles as those governing the placement of open laparotomy incisions. We recommend that the two lateral portals are inserted lateral to the inferior epigastric vessels. We attempt not only to avoid these vessels but also to ensure that the trocars are inserted laterally to the rectus muscle (Fig. 4.12). This location allows the trocar to pass through the less well-defined

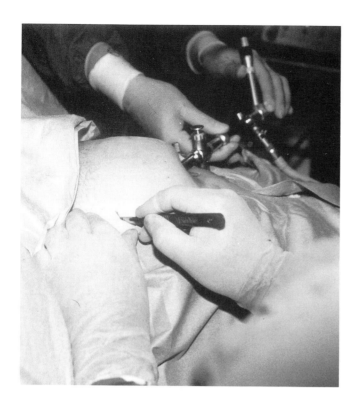

Fig. 4.12 Incision for left lower trocar placement. Lateral to rectus muscle and two finger breadths above the symphysis pubis.

external and internal oblique muscles. This situation makes the removal and reinsertion of trocars a simpler procedure, particularly if the trocar is inserted at right angles to the skin, thus reducing to a minimum the tissue penetrated (Fig. 4.13).

The inferior epigastric arteries, which ascend from the round ligament, may be damaged during insertion of these lateral trocars. Great care must be taken to avoid them when the trocars are inserted. They

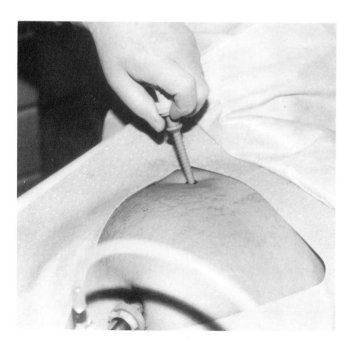

Fig. 4.13 Insertion of trocar at right-angles to skin.

are traditionally located by a transillumination technique. The distal tip of the laparoscope and its associated bright light source are placed in contact with the parietal peritoneum (Fig. 4.14). In thinner patients, vessels can be identified but these are often only superficial veins, and, in more obese patients, these vessels usually cannot be shown. Reich has described a more reliable way of defining the course of the inferior epigastric vessels. These arteries are known to lie between and just above two veins. These venae comitantes can almost invariably be found on direct laparoscopic inspection lateral to the obliterated umbilical artery, around which they curve. If the trocar is inserted laterally to these venae comitantes, the inferior epigastric artery will usually be safe.

Recommendation

The lateral secondary trocars should be inserted in the left and right iliac fossae, at a variable distance above the symphysis pubi but always lateral to the inferior epigastric artery and also lateral to the bulk of the rectus muscle.

Secondary trocars

Trocars of 5 mm diameter are adequate for most laparoscopic procedures. If, however, it is anticipated that cannulae of 10 or 12 mm diameter will be required at some stage, it is preferable to insert the larger size at the beginning of the operation and then use reducing sleeves or valves to accommodate the smaller instruments. An increasing number of designs of trocars are now available. The type most gynaecologists are familiar

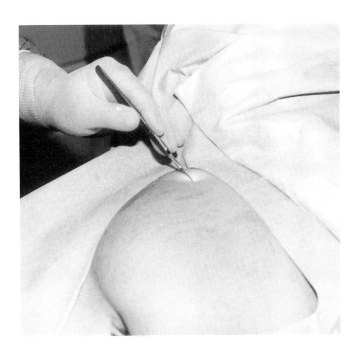

Fig. 4.14 Transillumination to demonstrate superficial vessels prior to incision.

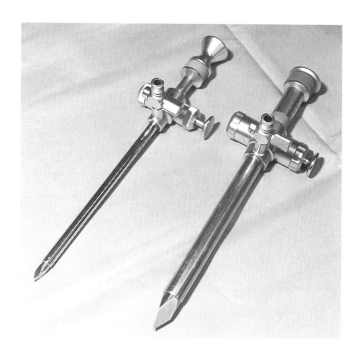

Fig. 4.15 5- and 10-mm reusable trumpet valve trocars.

with is the 5- or 10-mm reusable stainless-steel device with a trumpet valve and insufflation port (Fig. 4.15). These time-honoured devices give a good airtight seal around instruments but when the trumpet piston is released the instrument is compressed and difficult to move. An assistant must be available to open the valve every time it is necessary to reposition the instrument. This is both inefficient and inconvenient and this design cannot be recommended. The trumpet valve in this design of instrument is forced closed with a spring. Dr Alan Johns recommends that this spring is removed and he finds that then the friction between the trocar and the instrument it contains is dramatically reduced.

The only function of the secondary trocars is to act as a conduit to permit the insertion of instruments. Valves are placed in trocars to prevent loss of the pneumatoperitoneum but all valves impair the primary function of the trocar, which is to facilitate the rapid intro-duction and removal of instruments (see Fig. 3.16). The optimum secondary-puncture trocar valve should not obstruct the passage of the instruments. Many trocars are too long and often slip so that the whole barrel comes to lie in the abdominal cavity. In this position it is often difficult to push a forceps or stapling device far enough out of the cannula barrel to permit proper opening of the device. A short cannula, just long enough to comfortably enter the abdominal cavity, fitted with simple flap valves is to be preferred. Apple Medical (Bolton, MA) make an all-plastic sheath model (see Figs 3.15 and 4.16) and R. Wolfe (Rosemont, IL) make a similar all-stainless-steel model.

Straight trocar sheaths not only readily slip down to their full length inside the cavity but can also easily be inadvertently removed

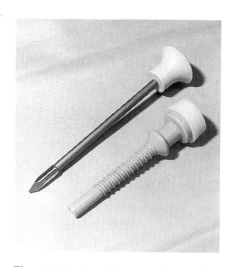

Fig. 4.16 An Apple trocar with securing screw threads.

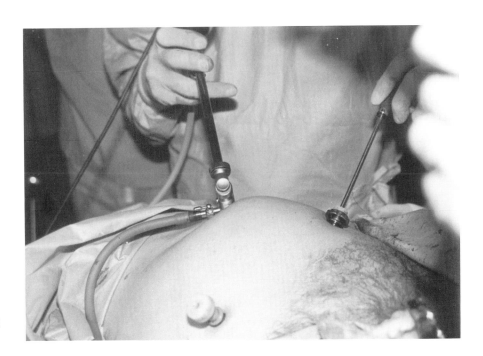

Fig. 4.17 Umbilical and two lower lateral trocars in position.

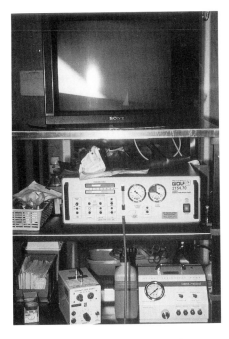

Fig. 4.18 A large equipment stack containing surgeon's video monitor (top), electronic CO_2 insufflator (middle) and irrigation equipment (bottom).

from the cavity when the instruments are pulled out. Screw threads, either permanent or as an additional accessory which can be secured to the trocar outer sheath, are useful (Fig. 4.16). These screw threads can be used to hold the sleeve firmly in the fascia at the optimum height. The Dexide trocar fixes the trocar in the optimum position in a novel manner, as described in Chapter 3 (see Fig. 3.14).

It is recommended that second- and third-entry-portal trocars should be inserted at right angles to the skin to make removal and reinsertion of the whole cannula as easy as possible. The intended site of emergence of the trocar can be determined by depressing the abdominal wall with the handle of a scalpel and observing the site internally with the laparoscope. When the correct position is chosen, the laparoscope should be positioned so that the tip of the trocar can be seen to emerge from the abdominal wall and can under direct vision be guided to a safe and satisfactory position. When this technique is used, expensive spring-loaded protective sheaths are not necessary and are not recommended.

When the trocars are all satisfactorily positioned (Fig. 4.17), the remainder of the supportive equipment must be assembled in a methodical manner (Fig. 4.18). A considerable quantity of electronic equipment is required for this type of surgery and it is helpful if this is collected together in space-saving stacking towers. An equipment stack with the surgeon's video-monitor, the CO_2 insufflator and the irrigation equipment should be placed on the opposite side of the patient and angled to the surgeon at the most convenient angle for him/her. A second equipment stack is placed behind the surgeon and angled so that his/her nurse and assistant may get an optimum view. This stack can contain the light source, camera control unit and video-recorder but obviously these arrangements may be varied to suit local conditions and equipment. What is important is that all the equipment is stored in as convenient, logical and compact a manner as possible, for space around the patient soon becomes at a premium in this type of surgery. Care should be taken to ensure that gas and fluid lines and electrical cables are arranged in such a way as to avoid the possibility of confusion or danger. Once everything is connected, the video-camera and the light cable are attached to the laparoscope and the procedure then always begins with a thorough inspection of the whole abdominal cavity and pelvis.

Recommendation

Short, straight, 5-mm sleeves with a simple flap-valve system, integral screw threads and sharp trocar points are recommended.

Suction and irrigation systems: aquadissection

One of the most important of all instruments for effective laparoscopic instruments is an effective suction–irrigation system. These systems will remove blood, peritoneal fluid and debris from the cavity and the operative site can be bathed and cleansed with irrigation fluids to maintain an optimum view at all times. The hydraulic energy from the pressurized fluid source can also be used as a most effective dissector. This process of aquadissection is particularly useful as the force it can exert is multidirectional and is therefore more effective than a unidirectional one, such as blunt probing, in opening up cleavage planes. Such a system transmits the fluid down lines of least tissue resistance and therefore opens up the tissues in the most correct anatomical planes.

It is recommended that the aquadissector should have a single large channel down which the suction and aspiration functions can be performed alternately. Devices with separate suction and irrigation channels side by side are less effective because they have significantly less suction and irrigation capacity than a single-channel probe of similar diameter. Reich prefers an aquadissector with no perforations at the distal end so that it can also be used in the suction mode as a suction retractor. Johns recommends that there should be two perforations of fairly large size about 5 mm from the distal tip of the probe to increase the lateral dissecting potential. Multiple small perforations favoured by some manufacturers appear to have little function.

The simplest design of suction–irrigation probe consists of a hollow tube with a three-way tap on the proximal end. One arm of this tap can be connected to the standard theatre suction system via a series of graduated collecting bottles. The other arm of the tap can be connected to the fluid infusion system. A variation of this design is the Semm monofilar-bivalent irrigation cannula, which consists of an oblong metal

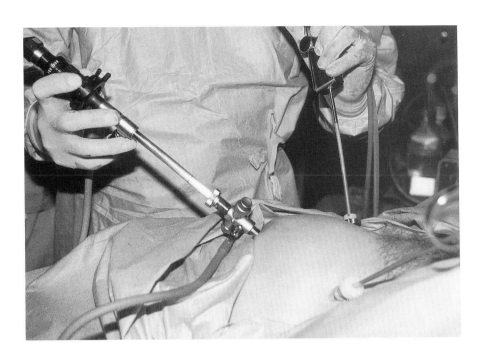

Fig. 4.19 Irrigation and suction cannula with large button controls.

control panel at the proximal end with separate irrigation and suction inputs and large staple control buttons (Fig. 4.19). A third commonly used variant of the irrigation cannula is the Nezhat cannula. This hollow tube has two trumpet valves to control suction and irrigation functions.

Fluid must be pumped into and out of the cavity. The simplest fluid pump is to suspend the soft infusion bag from a pole and wrap a blood-pressure cuff around this. Satisfactory flow rates can be achieved with this system. Garry has recently used a pressure bag sufficiently large to surround a 3-litre bag of infusion fluid. Two of these, connected by Y-shaped tubing, provide an almost unlimited quantity of fluid at a reasonable rate. The first specifically designed suction−irrigation device was the Semm Aqua-Purator (Fig. 4.20) (Wisap, Sauerlach, Germany).

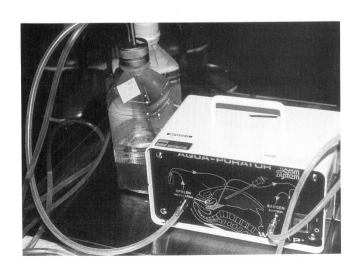

Fig. 4.20 A Semm Aqua-Purator irrigation system.

This device pumps warmed fluid at a rate of 250 ml every 10 seconds. The Nezhat pump or Nezhat Dorsey pump, a device powered by pressurized CO_2 gas, with two irrigation bottles connected so that a continuous flow of fluid can be maintained, has also been introduced (Fig. 4.21) (Cabot Medical, Langthorne, PA, and K. Storz, Tüttlingen, Germany).

Other varieties of suction–irrigators have been developed and they include disposable systems such as the Irrivac (Baxter-Travenol), in which the pressure is controlled and varied by pushing on an automatically filling vacuum bulb or syringe in the system. These systems are convenient but less effective and more costly than the reusable systems. A pulsatile water-jet irrigator, the Simpulse with endo-flow irrigation system (Davol, Cranston, RI), makes use of compressed nitrogen at 80 p.s.i. to generate high-pressure liquid pulsations which can produce efficient aquadissection.

Aquadissection may also be achieved with ultrasonic dissectors (Valleylab, Olympus). These devices vibrate very rapidly at 23 kHz frequency with adjustable amplitude up to 350 μm. The vibrations induced can selectively fragment soft, firm and even tough fibrous tissue. Such devices have suction, irrigation, cutting and coagulation capabilities.

For suction, a closed collection system such as the Medi-Vac CRD suction system (Baxter), with four 3000-ml canisters mounted on a carousel and hooked to wall suction at negative pressure of 200 mmHg, is very satisfactory.

Recommendation

A first-rate suction–irrigation system capable of delivering and removing large volumes of fluid rapidly is essential for operative laparoscopy. The Semm Aqua-Purator and the Nezhat hydrodissection

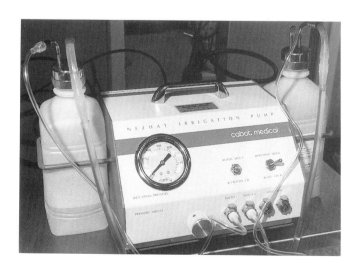

Fig. 4.21 A Nezhat irrigation pump.

system are well-tried systems which can be recommended. The hydro-dissector should have a single channel with only two or no lateral irrigation holes.

Forceps

There are now so many types and makes of laparoscopic forceps available that the newcomer to the field must inevitably be intimidated by the choice available (Fig. 4.22). Essentially, however, an adequate complement of atraumatic and toothed, blunt-nosed and needle-pointed, straight and curved shapes is required. This is identical to the requirements for open surgery and the type of instruments required for the classical procedure should, as far as possible, be replicated laparoscopically. The types of forceps available are fully described in Chapter 3. Each pattern is available in reusable stainless steel or disposable form. In all units with access to adequate sterilization facilities, the authors can find no reason for preferring the inferior quality and greater expense of disposable forceps and recommend the purchase of well-made reusable alternatives whenever possible.

Self-retaining, atraumatic forceps are the 'retractors' of operative laparoscopy, maintaining exposure and position. They are used in conjunction with a uterine manipulator to produce counter-traction and tissue tension, which is so essential to surgery of any nature. Only this type of forceps should be used on tissue to be retained. At least two types of atraumatic forceps should be available. Blunt, round-nose forceps are required to displace bowel and grasp some pelvic structures (Fig. 4.23). Stronger atraumatic or multipronged forceps are

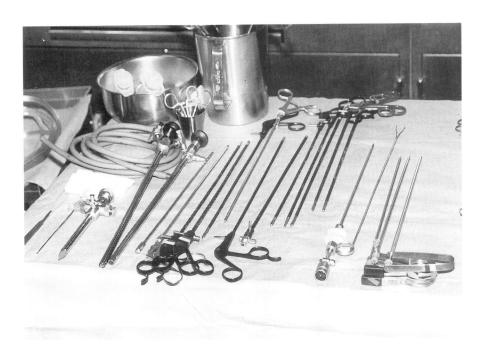

Fig. 4.22 Selection of forceps and associated equipment required for advanced laparoscopic surgery.

required to stabilize the ovaries and other mobile structures to be conserved (see Fig. 3.20). Dissection of the ureters requires smooth- or rounded-tip atraumatic grasping forceps (Fig. 4.24). Petlin 45° and 90° curved dissecting forceps are useful for dissecting out and particularly for getting behind vascular and tubular pedicles (Fig. 4.25).

For tissues to be removed, particularly when it is essential to maintain traction, forceps with single or multiple teeth should be available (Fig. 4.26). If the structure to be removed is a fibroid or similar mass, it can often best be secured and mobilized with myoma drills or corkscrews. These can be useful when considerable traction is required.

For most laparoscopic surgery the 5-mm-size instrument is the preferred size. Some instruments can also be usefully employed in the smaller 3-mm size and the larger 10-mm instruments, particularly the large claw-shaped tooth forceps and the spoon-shaped grasping forceps, may be useful (Fig. 4.27). Semm now recommends 15- and 20-mm-diameter macromorcellator instruments but these sized instruments are seldom used by other endoscopic surgeons as yet.

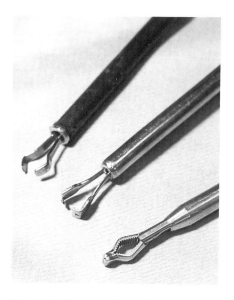

Fig. 4.23 Close up of round grasping forceps.

Recommendation

A variety of well-made stainless-steel reusable 5-mm atraumatic and toothed dissecting and grasping forceps are required for effective laparoscopic surgery. Some 10-mm- and perhaps larger-diameter instruments may also occasionally be required.

Scissors

Laparoscopic scissors can be the most frustrating of all endoscopic instruments because it seems to be very difficult to keep them sharp and therefore useful. Most laparoscopic scissors have one movable and one fixed blade. This design may have been easier to adapt for laparoscopic use but most surgeons are more used to, and more comfortable with, scissors in which both blades open and close. At least four types of scissors are required for comprehensive laparoscopic surgery (Fig. 3.26 and Fig. 4.28):

1 Hook-shaped scissors with rounded points and either smooth or serrated blades. These scissors are the laparoscopic equivalent of the Mayo's scissors and are used to cut relatively thick tissues and also for cutting sutures.

2 Curved scissors with rounded tips and smooth blades. These are the laparoscopic equivalents of 'Metzenbaum' scissors and are used for the same type of general dissection work.

3 Flat scissors with rounded ends are often called peritoneal scissors and are of particular value in cutting thinner structures such as the peritoneum and in forming the bladder flap.

4 Microscissors have needle-shaped points and small sharp blades.

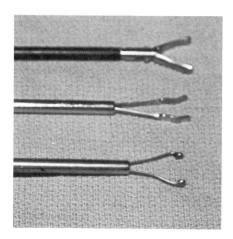

Fig. 4.24 Further selection of atraumatic forceps.

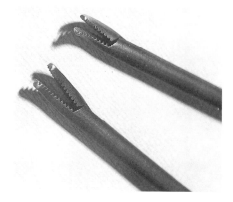

Fig. 4.25 Petlin 45° and 90° curved dissecting forceps.

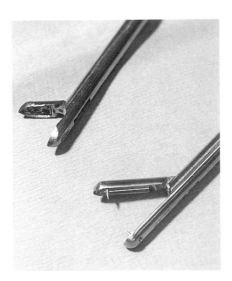

Fig. 4.26 5-mm biopsy forceps. The single-toothed version is an excellent grasping forceps.

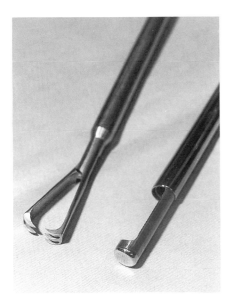

Fig. 4.27 10-mm toothed grasping forcep (left).

These are used for fine dissection work, for example with tubal surgery. The points of these scissors are sharp and they must be handled with particular care to avoid damage to the viscera during insertion and movement around the cavity.

Most of these designs are again available in both reusable and disposable forms. Because of the difficulties encountered in maintaining the sharp cutting edge of most laparoscopic scissors, the extra costs of the disposable equipment may well be justified. We have found the Endo-Shear (AutoSuture/USSC) to be particularly useful curved scissors.

Recommendation

Several different patterns of sharp 5-mm scissors are required for laparoscopic surgery. These may be reusable or disposable, depending on preference and budget.

Electrosurgical techniques

The principles of the use of electrosurgical equipment in laparoscopic surgery have been discussed in Chapter 3. The authors consider that the use of electrosurgical techniques to produce large-vessel haemostasis is the corner-stone of some advanced laparoscopic techniques, including laparoscopic hysterectomy.

Cutting is best achieved with unmodulated cutting current combined with a 1-mm needle-, 3-mm knife- or other-shaped but thin-edged electrode. The nature of the effect of the current can be modified by the shape of the electrode used. Hook-, button-, spatula- and spoon-shaped electrodes may be used in this manner (Fig. 4.29). If the sharp edge of a spoon-shaped electrode is applied to the tissue, a cutting effect will be produced, but, if the same cutting current is applied with the broad spoon face, a coagulation effect will be produced.

Cutting and coagulation of small and moderate-sized blood-vessels

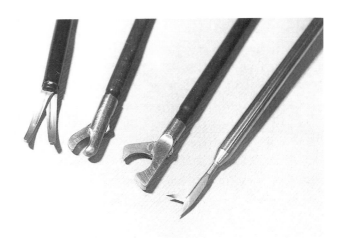

Fig. 4.28 Selection of laparoscopic scissors.

can be performed in an almost simultaneous process, using cutting unipolar current and insulated scissors. The blades of the scissors are first held slightly apart with the small-vessel-containing tissue between. In this position, the cutting current will produce a significant coagulation effect. Following this, the blades of the scissors can be closed and the tissues divided in a simple mechanical manner.

Larger vessels, including the ovarian and uterine arteries, cannot be successfully occluded in this way, but Reich and others have clearly shown that bipolar diathermy can desiccate and effectively occlude vessels of this calibre (Fig. 4.30). To be successful it is important that the blades of the bipolar forceps are correctly applied for the optimum time. If too high a current is used, the outside of the pedicle will coagulate rapidly but the vessel in the centre may not be affected. If the current is maintained for too long, the vessel may be burnt through and occlusion will again not occur. If coagulation is excessive, the coagulum may stick to the forceps and be torn away with the instrument, again failing to produce haemostasis. To effectively use this technique, it is important to measure the flow of current and continue desiccation until the current ceases to flow. This can be detected either by connecting a current flowmeter into the system and continuing to activate the pedal until the current stops flowing or, better, by computing this automatically, using the automatic cutting and coagulation system of the Erbe electrosurgical equipment.

Excision of the ovary, the tube or the whole uterus may best be achieved using this technique of bipolar desiccation. Kleppinger bipolar forceps are used to take a series of small bites of the infundibulopelvic ligament. The tissues are completely desiccated and, when the current stops flowing, the desiccated tissue is divided with scissors or with an Nd-YAG laser with sapphire tips. Such an approach parallels good open-surgical technique when a haemostat (bipolar forceps) is first applied and the pedicle is then secured by suturing (desiccation) and then divided with a knife or scissors (scissors or laser). Too large a bite will lead to wide lateral spread of the current beyond the forceps tip, with the risk of damage to surrounding structures. Division should be close to the specimen side of the zone of coagulation so that the maximum amount of compressed and sealed vessels remain in the area of desiccation.

Vessels may also be coagulated using a cutting spray type of current. This technique is known as fulguration. If a highly modulated, intense current is applied through an electrode held a short distance above the tissue, the current will arc and in this process produce intense local coagulation. The distance this arc can be made to jump can be increased using an argon beam coagulator, in the manner described in Chapter 3.

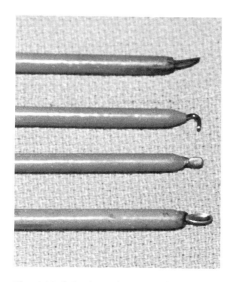

Fig. 4.29 Selection of monopolar laparoscopic tips.

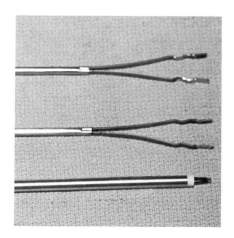

Fig. 4.30 Kleppinger (top and middle) and micro-bipolar forceps (bottom).

Recommendation

The authors consider a modern electrosurgical unit with both unipolar and bipolar facilities to be the most important single item of equipment necessary for safe laparoscopic surgery.

Lasers in laparoscopic surgery

The principles and tissue effects of various lasers have been discussed in the previous chapter. The CO_2 beam or a fibre laser directed down the 5-mm working channel of a 10-mm operating hysteroscope converts the umbilical incision into a portal for surgery, thereby reducing the need for an additional portal of entry.

The CO_2 beam directed via a Nezhat type of direct coupler produces tissue vaporization (see Fig. 3.8). This can be used to produce vaporization of lesions such as deposits of endometriosis but is more often used for division of tissues, separation of adhesions and excision of tissue in the manner of scissors. Small blood-vessels may be coagulated with this modality but continued use during significant bleeding usually results in 'burnt black blood' but no haemostasis.

The major advantage of the CO_2 wavelength is that, as it is totally absorbed by intracellular water, the laser energy is rapidly converted to thermal energy and the volume of tissue penetrated is no more than 0.1 mm. This results in more precise cutting and greater safety than can be achieved with electrosurgery or other laser modalities. This property is of particular value when working close to vital structures, particularly when dissecting the ureter and the pelvic side-wall. The precision of the incision and the amount of tissue damage is further reduced when superpulse or ultrapulse modalities are used. These alternate relatively short bursts of high-powered laser energy with long periods of inactivity, which result in rapid tissue cooling; this reduces heat conduction and minimizes subsequent tissue damage.

The fibre-laser wavelengths penetrate tissue more deeply and produce more lateral tissue damage but also more tissue coagulation. Because of the lateral tissue coagulation, the incision produced by such lasers is less precise but more haemostatic than that associated with the CO_2 laser. The deep lateral tissue damage associated with the use of the bare-fibre Nd-YAG laser can be minimized by using appropriately shaped sapphire probes (Fig. 4.31). These probes concentrate the energy and provide very high-power densities exactly where they are needed, at the tip of the probe. In such a configuration the power density drops off rapidly within a short distance of the sapphire tip, giving a 'what you see is what you get' type of incision similar to that produced by the CO_2 wavelength but with more haemostatic effect. The semirigid handpiece used with this equipment gives contact and a tissue feel which is preferred by some surgeons (Figs 4.32 and 4.33). These advan-

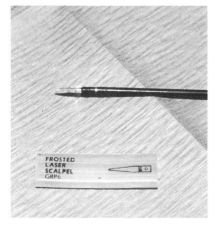

Fig. 4.31 Laparoscopic handpiece with frosted scalpel type of sapphire tip.

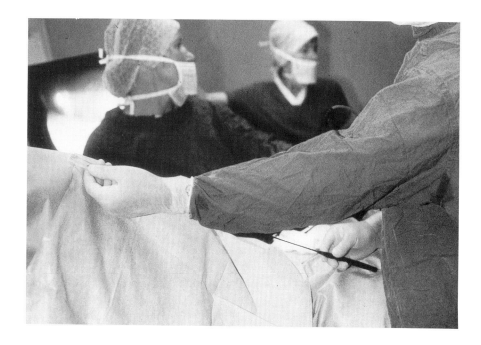

Fig. 4.32 Attaching a sapphire tip to a laparoscopic handpiece.

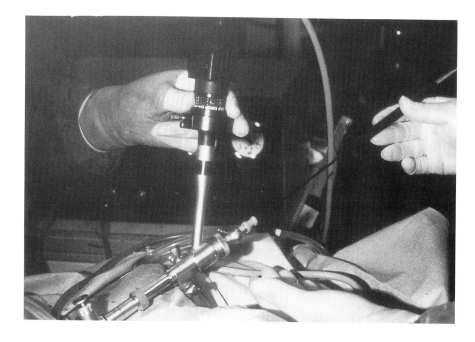

Fig. 4.33 Nd-YAG laser fibre inserted down operating channel of the laparoscope.

tages are offset by the considerable costs of the sapphire probes and handpieces.

The tips become very hot and must be cooled by a medium that is forced down a coaxial channel. If CO_2 gas is used as the coolant, the maximum laser power should be 15 W and, if the tip is cooled with liquid, 15–18 W may be required. It is important to ensure that only the tip of the probe is used to cut tissue and that as far as possible it is held at right angles to the tissue to be divided. The optimum cutting effect is then obtained by moving the tip back and forth so that it only gently slides over the surface of the tissue. Only the tip of the probe delivers the laser energy and if the surgeon tries to use the probe in the same way as an electrosurgical blade, using the sides of the device, poor results will be obtained. With good technique, precise cutting with simultaneous coagulation can be produced with the Nd-YAG wavelength.

As a contact technique, there is less risk of 'past-pointing' tissue damage and, because of its different effect on tissue, it produces less smoke than either electrosurgery or CO_2 laser modalities. This may be a significant advantage in the close confines of the abdominal cavity, where it is important to ensure excellent vision at all times, particularly at times when haemostasis might be a problem. This modality may be used for division of vascular and avascular adhesions, for dividing the uterovesical peritoneum and forming the bladder flap during laparoscopic hysterectomy. If anterior and posterior colpotomies and division of the uterosacral ligaments are to be performed, the Nd-YAG laser and sapphire tip system will perform this with less bleeding and smoke production than with the CO_2 laser and with less unwanted tissue destruction and smoke production than with electrosurgery. These potential advantages are offset by the much greater costs of the disposables.

Recommendation

Lasers are not essential for operative laparoscopy and many surgeons can achieve excellent results without them. The authors, however, believe that lasers have properties which complement other modalities and in some circumstances can be the most convenient and effective method of dissecting and removing tissue without blood loss. A CO_2 laser should have a superpulse or ultrapulse mode and should be delivered via a direct coupler to the laparoscope or secondary trocar. This wavelength's main advantage is its ability to produce very precise cutting with minimal tissue damage. The fibre lasers, particularly the Nd-YAG laser wavelength, should be delivered via a sapphire or sculptured tip and this configuration can provide fairly accurate cutting with considerable associated haemostatic effect. This is a more expensive modality but provides tissue feel and is associated with less smoke production than other systems.

Suturing techniques

Nothing increases the potential scope of laparoscopic surgery more than the acquisition of the ability to confidently tie surgical knots down the laparoscope. The aim of all laparoscopic suture techniques is to ligate major blood-vessels and tissue pedicles with the same degree of security as would be acceptable at open surgery. Achieving this aim is not easy and requires considerable experimentation and practice. Various approaches have been adopted and these will now be described in detail.

Endoloop system

Perhaps the simplest of the systems to learn is the Ethicon 'endoloop' system. This technique, described and popularized by Semm [3], can be used for controlling mobile pedicles and vessels which have already been divided and also for closing openings in cystic structures. The system consists of a pre-tied Roeder loop attached to a plastic shaft (Fig. 4.34). One end of the suture passes up the centre of the shaft and is attached to the proximal end. This end can be broken and pulled to tighten the knot. The unbroken shaft and large 'lasso' knot are back-loaded into a 3-mm introducing sleeve until the loop is completely inside the barrel. The assembled introducer is then inserted down a 5-mm trocar into the abdominal cavity. The shaft is then advanced and the exposed loop positioned around the tissue to be ligated. The position of tissue and loop may be adjusted with the contralateral grasping forceps. When correctly positioned, the tissue or pedicle is pulled up through the loop, which is then tightened by breaking the shaft at the red band. The small end is pulled backwards whilst simultaneously sliding the plastic shaft forwards to the intended position of the ligature. This movement allows the knot to slide forward as the loop decreases in size. The plastic shaft pushes the knot home and the final tightening is achieved by pulling the snapped-off end of the ligature firmly. Once the knot is secured, the plastic shaft is drawn into the introducer away from the knot. The ligature is then cut by removing the grasping forceps and replacing it with 5-mm hooked scissors and cutting about 5 mm from the knot.

Extracorporeal endosuture system

When it is necessary to pass the suture through tissue before tying it, the Ethicon endoknot system may be used. This consists of a plastic shaft, identical to that used in the endoloop system, attached to a length of suture material, usually chromic catgut, and a straight or ski-shaped atraumatic needle. This system can be used to ligate vessels, reconstruct organs, approximate opposing tissue surfaces and suture anastomoses.

The suture is grasped just below the swage point with a 3-mm needle-holder. The needle-holder is inserted into the introducer so that the suture bends and the needle can follow the introducer. The loaded trocar is then introduced into the cavity through a 5-mm trocar. A 5-mm grasper is inserted through the contralateral trocar. The needle is passed from the needle-holder to the grasper and, when steadied,

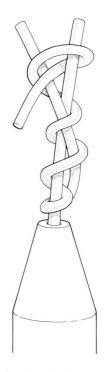

Fig. 4.34 Roeder slip knot.

repositioned in the needle-holder at the desired location. The needle may then be passed through the tissue and grasped as it emerges. The tip of the needle is then again gripped with the needle-holder and the suture pulled further through the tissue, with the grasper relieving tension on the suture line. The needle is released and the suture material is grasped below the swage point again and then drawn up through the trocar and removed from the abdominal cavity.

An assistant places his finger on the introducer channel to prevent excessive loss of gas. The needle is cut off and then a single throw is formed. A Roeder knot is then tied by holding the knot firmly between thumb and third finger. With the free end, a single loop is made around the suture and three more loops are made around both limbs of the loop. The tail of the suture is then inserted through the last loop to be formed (i.e. the one just above the assistant's finger) and the excess tail trimmed. When this Roeder's knot is satisfactorily formed, it can be tightened in the way described in the previous section. Semm has devised a rotating collar, which facilitates the production of such an extracorporeal Roeder knot [4].

Intracorporeal knot-tying

Using the same instruments, knots can be tied intracorporeally. The suture material is first cut to the desired length. If a straight needle is used, it is loaded into a 5-mm introducer in the same manner as described above. If a smaller curved needle is preferred, it is loaded into the larger 8-mm introducer in the following way. The 5-mm needle-holder is passed through the introducer and the tail of the suture is grasped. The entire length of the suture is then pulled back through the introducer, leaving only the needle hanging free. The tail of the suture is released and the needle-holder reinserted down the length of the introducer, grasping the swage point. Care must be taken to keep the needle curve parallel to the needle-holder as the needle is pulled into the distal end of the introducer. The loaded introducer is inserted down a 10-mm trocar.

Once in the cavity, either type of needle is picked up with the contralateral grasper, steadied and then regrasped in the correct position with the needle-holder and passed through the tissue. The remaining length of suture is brought into the cavity and the strands are equalized on either side of the structure to be ligated. The needle may be removed or retained at this stage. The suture is wrapped twice around the needle-holder, which is held steady, keeping the swage of the needle, if still attached, pointing towards the needle-holder. With the free grasper, the end of the suture should then be removed from the jaws of the needle-holder. The looped needle-holder should then pick up the remaining free end of the suture and each tail should be pulled in an opposite direction to form the first throw of the knot. The procedure should then be repeated and the knot tightened.

Simplified method for ligating

A simple technique using a knot-pusher for laparoscopic suturing was described by Dr Cortney Clarke in 1972 [5]. This technique appears to have been forgotten for some years until rediscovered and published by Reich in 1992 [6]. It is a technique that greatly simplifies laparoscopic suturing and is more rapid and convenient to perform than any of the methods described above.

To suture with a straight needle, the needle is grasped behind the swage point and introduced down a short trocar sheath with no or minimal trap. When picked up, the needle is passed through the tissues and then is regrasped and removed through the same trocar. The needle is cut and both strands are grasped in the surgeon's left hand after making a simple half-hitch. The Clarke—Reich knot-pusher (Marlow Surgical) is put on the suture, which is held firm across the index finger. The throw is then pushed rapidly down to the tissue. A square knot is made by making a second half-hitch and again pushing this down to the tissue with the knot-pusher. This secures the knot whilst tension is maintained from above. Suture-tying outside the peritoneal cavity is made easier by using trocars without trumpet valves.

Most surgeons prefer curved needles, as they are easier to place accurately. The techniques previously described can only use straight, ski-shaped or small-diameter curved needles. Reich has recently described a simple technique in which any reasonably sized needle can be inserted into the abdominal cavity through a 5-mm secondary-puncture incision (Fig. 4.35) [6].

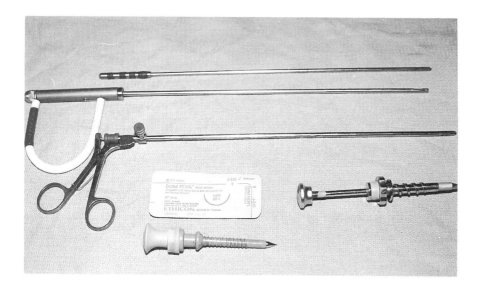

Fig. 4.35 Equipment required for extracorporeal knot tying with Reich's technique.

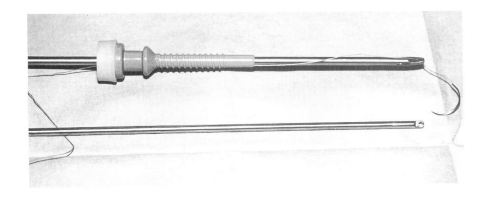

Fig. 4.36 A trocar sleeve loaded for insertion of curved needle into the abdominal cavity.

For this technique it is important to ensure that the lower-quadrant secondary-puncture incisions are inserted lateral to the thick rectus muscle. The trocar should also be inserted vertically and at right angles to the skin, to ensure the creation of an obvious straight tract down the shortest distance into the cavity. If a larger needle, such as a CT 1, is required, the left 5-mm trocar sleeve is removed and an assistant places a finger over the incision to prevent the loss of the pneumatoperitoneum. The distal end of the suture is picked up with a needle-holder and back-loaded through the trocar sleeve. The needle-holder is then reinserted into the sleeve and the suture is regrasped 2–4 cm from the swage (Fig. 4.36). The needle-holder is then inserted down the tract into the cavity, pulling the needle behind. Once the needle is inside the cavity, the trocar is reinserted over the needle-holder down the same tract (Fig. 4.37). The needle is dropped, positioned and regrasped.

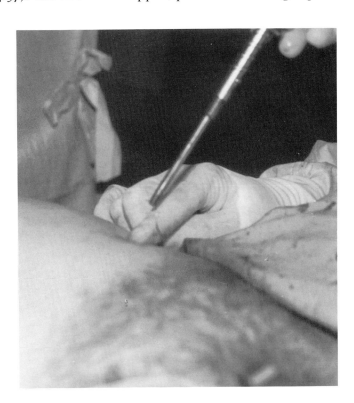

Fig. 4.37 The curved needle about to be inserted into the abdominal cavity.

This is the most difficult part of this procedure. When it is correctly orientated in the needle-holder, it is pushed through the desired tissues. More of the suture is pulled through the tissue and then the needle and about 3 cm of suture are cut free. The needle is temporarily stored in the cavity or inserted into the abdominal wall in a convenient location. The free end of the suture is then picked up with the needle-holder and pulled up through the trocar sleeve. An extracorporeal half-hitch is formed and pushed down to the operative site with the knot-pusher (Fig. 4.38). A second hitch is also pushed firmly down on to the first throw and the knot tightened (Fig. 4.39). The needle is removed by grasping the remaining tail and pulling it out of the trocar tract, after first removing the cannula above skin level.

Recommendation

The ability to tie secure knots laparoscopically is an important skill which increases the confidence and range of procedures which a surgeon can tackle laparoscopically. The extracorporeal technique of Clarke and Reich is strongly recommended as the most convenient and effective of the alternatives currently available, for it can be used with almost any needle and any suture material in almost any situation.

Staples

Another effective method for securing haemostasis is with metal or

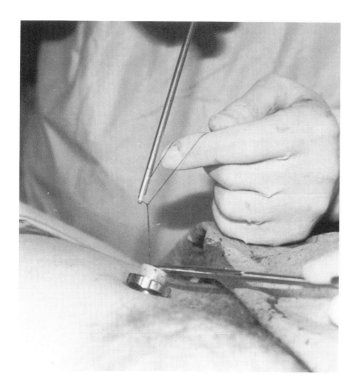

Fig. 4.38 The half hitch of the knot being pushed into the abdominal cavity.

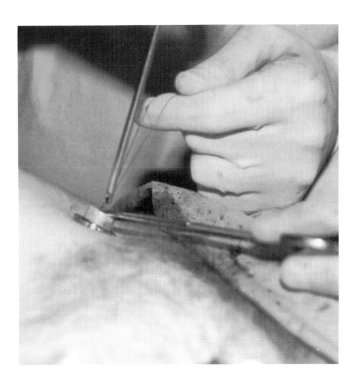

Fig. 4.39 A second hitch pushed down to tighten the knot.

absorbable staples. They can be used to produce large-vessel haemostasis during hysterectomy. Single, inert, non-reactive titanium clips can be placed on the bleeding vessel with a reusable stainless-steel laparoscopic applicator. It is always inconvenient, often troublesome and sometimes dangerous to remove the applicator from the cavity with a major vessel incompletely sealed. To overcome this disadvantage AutoSuture/USSC (Endo Clip) and Ethicon (Ligaclip) have produced disposable automatic clip applicators (see Fig. 3.27). Each cartridge contains 20 staples, which are inserted down a 10-mm trocar. It is necessary to skeletonize the vessels before these staples are applied.

More effective haemostasis may be obtained with the Multi-fire Endo GIA 30 stapling device (AutoSuture/USSC). This device is inserted down a 12-mm cannula and consists of a handle, a shaft and an anvil which can be used for up to four applications. To fire against this anvil, there is a single-use stapling cartridge containing six layers of titanium staples and a self-contained knife blade (Fig. 4.40). The staples

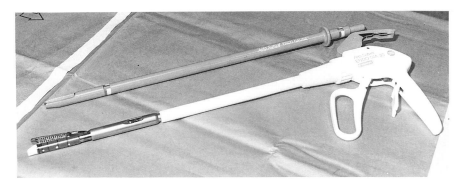

Fig. 4.40 An autoSuture Endo GIA 30 staple gun with stapling cartridge (bottom) and an Endo gauge measuring rod (above).

are arranged so that three rows lie on each side of the divided tissue.
The outer and inner rows of each group are parallel and the middle
row overlaps the spaces. Such an arrangement should occlude all vessels
passing through the stapled zone. Two types of cartridge are available:
the standard blue-tipped cartridge occludes to 1.5 mm and the white-
tipped vascular cartridge compresses to 1 mm.

The tissue to be divided is first measured by inserting an Endo
gauge down the 12-mm sleeve and placing it over the area to be
divided. This not only assesses that the tissue is of an appropriate
thickness for division with the Endo GIA and determines the optimum
cartridge to use but also allows the optimum angle of approach to be
determined. The gauge is removed and replaced by an applicator with
a suitable cartridge. Care must be taken to ensure that the jaws of
the stapler are below the cannula and completely free before opening
the device. The jaws are opened by fully elevating the grey lever on the
handle (Fig. 4.41). They are then manoeuvred into the desired position
and the jaws closed again by depressing the handle (Fig. 4.42). In this
position the tissues are held firmly between the cartridge and the anvil
but the staples have not been fired. The position of the jaws is checked
to ensure that no unintended important structures are included in the
bite. Only when this has been confirmed is the safety guard disengaged
and the handles brought together to fire the staples (Fig. 4.43). This
action applies the six rows of staples and simultaneously divides
the tissues. The staple line extends a little further than the incision.
The grey handle is again elevated, opening the jaws and allowing the
divided tissue to be disengaged. The dual staple lines must be carefully
inspected to ensure that haemostasis is secured. Persistent bleeding,

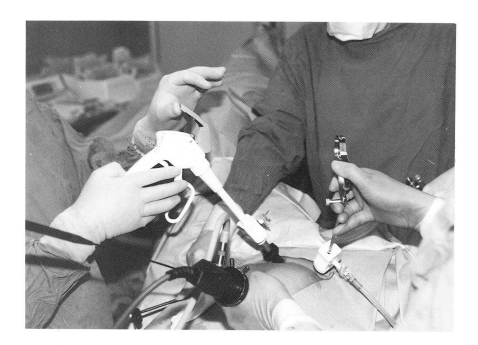

Fig. 4.41 Opening the jaws of the stapling cartridge with the grey opening lever.

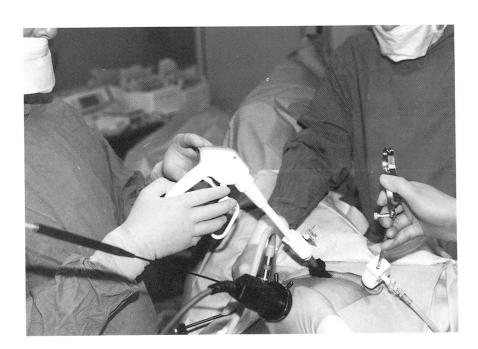

Fig. 4.42 Closing the jaws of the staple cartridge by depressing the handle.

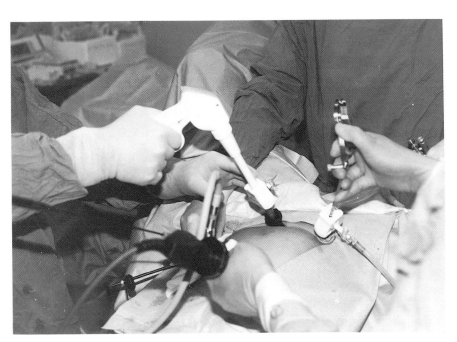

Fig. 4.43 Firing the instrument by closing the handles.

perhaps manifesting itself as a retroperitoneal haematoma, may occur if the device is not correctly applied.

During laparoscopic hysterectomy, the Endo GIA can be effectively applied to the infundibulopelvic ligaments and ovarian vessel. The staples are particularly advantageous and time-saving for application in a single bite to the round ligament, the tube and the utero-ovarian ligament. If the Endo GIA is to be applied to the uterine artery, the ureter must be dissected and demonstrated to lie clear before firing.

The authors do not recommend the Endo GIA in this situation, for the risk here of unintended ureteric damage is significant.

Recommendation

Endo GIA 30 staples are a rapid, effective and convenient method of securing major pedicles during laparoscopic hysterectomy. They are, however, expensive and should be used only with extreme care in the region of the ureter.

References

1 Hasson HM. Open laparoscopy vs. closed laparoscopy: a comparison of complication rates. *Adv Planned Parenthood* 1978; **13**: 41−50.
2 Semm K. Sicht kontrollierte peritoneum Perforation zur operativen Pelviskopie. *Geburtsh u. Frauenheilk* 1988; **48**: 436−439.
3 Semm K. Operative pelviscopy. *Br Med Bull* 1986; **42**: 284−295.
4 Semm K. Tissue-puncher and loop ligation: new aids for surgical therapeutic pelviscopy (laparoscopy) = endoscopic intra-abdominal surgery. *Endoscopy* 1978; **10**: 119−124.
5 Clarke HC. Laparoscopy − new instruments for suturing and ligation. *Fertil Steril* 1972; **23**: 274−277.
6 Reich H, Clarke HC, Sekel L. A simple method for ligating in operative laparoscopy with straight and curved needles. *Obstet Gynecol* 1992; **79**: 143−147.

5: Laparoscopic Hysterectomy

Definitions

Laparoscopic techniques can be used to completely remove the uterus or to facilitate a vaginal hysterectomy. The laparoscopic division of all major uterine pedicles and supports can properly be termed laparoscopic hysterectomy (LH). Lesser degrees of laparoscopic surgery to aid the vaginal removal of the uterus can more accurately be described as laparoscopic assisted vaginal hysterectomy (LAVH). Reich considers that the laparoscopic dissection of the uterus must continue down to and include the laparoscopic ligation of the uterine artery for the procedure to be considered a laparoscopic hysterectomy. Johns and Diamond have suggested the following classification system to define the various stages of laparoscopic hysterectomy and laparoscopic-assisted vaginal hysterectomy:

Stage 0 Diagnostic laparoscopy performed but no laparoscopic surgery required before a vaginal hysterectomy.

Stage 1 Laparoscopic adhesiolysis or excision of endometriosis before vaginal hysterectomy.

Stage 2 Either one or both adnexa, including the infundibulopelvic ligaments, freed laparoscopically prior to vaginal hysterectomy.

Stage 3 Bladder dissected from the uterus laparoscopically prior to vaginal hysterectomy.

Stage 4 All of the above performed and then uterine arteries transected laparoscopically prior to vaginal dissection of the uterosacral and cardinal ligaments.

Stage 5 Anterior and/or posterior colpotomy and freeing of the whole uterus performed laparoscopically.

Following Reich's definition, stages 4 and 5 above would be examples of laparoscopic hysterectomy and stages 0–3 would be examples of laparoscopic-assisted vaginal hysterectomy.

Independently, Professor Bruhat's group in Clermont-Ferrand suggested a three-stage definition of laparoscopic hysterectomy [1]:

Type 1 The endosurgery is limited to the adnexa.

Type 2 The endosurgery includes the uterine vessels whilst the cardinal and uterosacral ligaments are ligated vaginally.

Type 3 The procedure in its entirety is carried out endoscopically, including opening the vaginal wall.

They suggest that type 2 and 3 procedures are true endosurgical hysterectomies and type 1 can only be considered a prelude to vaginal hysterectomy.

These three major authorities agree that the route by which the uterine artery is secured determines if the hysterectomy should be considered an LH or an LAVH. In addition to this fundamental division of the types of laparoscopic hysterectomy into LH and LAVH, there are now a number of additional approaches which can be adopted. Reich recommends the more extensive classification of laparoscopic hysterectomy described below. Some type of classification such as this must be agreed before results and complications can be compared between centres and before a fair level of remuneration can be agreed with the health insurers for procedures of vastly different complexity. Applying a couple of Endo GIA staples to a small mobile uterus and then performing a standard vaginal hysterectomy is obviously a different degree of complexity to performing a complete laparoscopic removal of a 20-week-size uterus containing fibroids and surrounded by extensive endometriosis. These differences will need to be borne in mind when comparing techniques and results. An agreed, fully descriptive classification is therefore required and we suggest the following.

The complete laparoscopic removal of the uterus from all its supports should be called total laparoscopic hysterectomy (TLH) to differentiate it from the procedure where the cardinal and uterosacral ligaments are secured vaginally after laparoscopically securing the uterine arteries, which should be called a laparoscopic hysterectomy (LH). Increasing interest is being shown in the concept of conserving the cervix and performing a subtotal or supracervical hysterectomy. Laparoscopic supracervical hysterectomy (LSH) may be performed as described in Chapter 9, when it will be termed an LSH, or according to the techniques described by Kurt Semm in Chapter 6, when the procedure will be called CASH (classic abdominal SEMM hysterectomy) where SEMM stands for serrated-edge macromorcellator.

More extensive types of laparoscopic hysterectomy have also recently been described for the treatment of certain gynaecological malignancies (Chapter 10). Laparoscopic hysterectomy with bilateral pelvic-node lymphadenectomy (LHL), with or without omentectomy, has been described, as has radical laparoscopic hysterectomy (RLH) of the Wertheim's type. The complete proposed classification of laparoscopic hysterectomy is thus:

1   Diagnostic laparoscopy with vaginal hysterectomy (VH; Fig. 5.1).
2   Laparoscopic vault suspension after vaginal hysterectomy.
3   Laparoscopic-assisted vaginal hysterectomy (LAVH; Fig. 5.2).
4   Laparoscopic hysterectomy (LH; Fig. 5.3).
5   Total laparoscopic hysterectomy (TLH; Fig. 5.4).
6   Laparoscopic supracervical hysterectomy (LSH or CASH; Fig. 5.5).
7   Laparoscopic hysterectomy with lymphadenectomy (LHL).
8   Laparoscopic hysterectomy with lymphadenectomy and omentectomy (LHL+O).
9   Radical laparoscopic hysterectomy (RLH; Fig. 5.6).

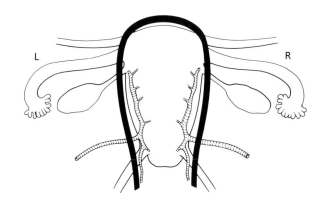

Fig. 5.1 Standard vaginal hysterectomy following a diagnostic laparoscopy.

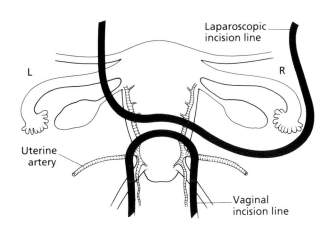

Fig. 5.2 Stage 3. Laparoscopic-assisted vaginal hysterectomy (LAVH) with laparoscopic mobilization of adnexa and securing of infundibulo-pelvic ligaments and vaginal securing of uterine arteries and uterosacral and cardinal ligaments.

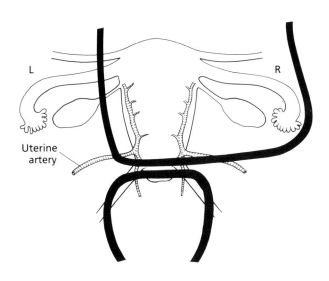

Fig. 5.3 Stage 4. Laparoscopic hysterectomy (LH). This stage includes laparoscopic division of uterine arteries but vaginal division of uterosacral and cardinal ligaments.

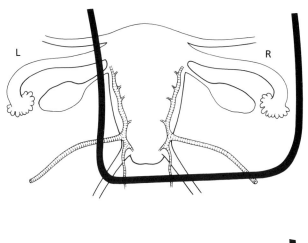

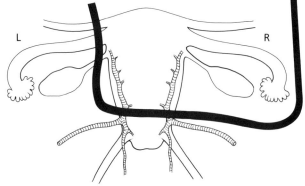

Fig. 5.4 Stage 5. Total laparoscopic hysterectomy (TLH). This stage involves the complete mobilization of the uterus laparoscopically including uterosacral and cardinal ligaments combined with laparoscopic opening of anterior and posterior cul-de-sacs.

Fig. 5.5 Stage 6. Laparoscopic supracervical hysterectomy (LSH). The adnexa and infundibulo-pelvic ligaments are mobilized laparoscopically and the uterine fundus is removed from the cervix at the level of the internal os.

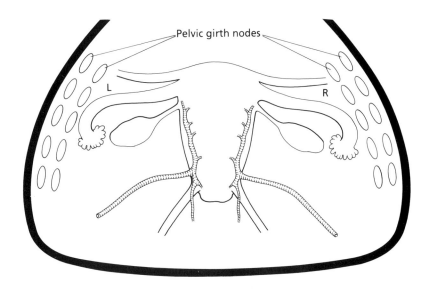

Fig. 5.6 Stage 9. Radical laparoscopic hysterectomy (RLH). A 'Wertheim's type of hysterectomy with full bilateral pelvic lymph node dissection and wide removal of adnexal tissue performed entirely with laparoscopic techniques.

These new procedures mean that the gynaecological textbooks must be rewritten, for there are now at least four methods of performing a standard hysterectomy and there are several subdivisions of these new categories. The main types of hysterectomy now available to the gynaecologist are:

1 Abdominal hysterectomy.

2   Laparoscopic hysterectomy.
3   Laparoscopic-assisted vaginal hysterectomy.
4   Vaginal hysterectomy.

Indications

The indications for laparoscopic hysterectomy and laparoscopic-assisted vaginal hysterectomy are not yet defined and each team involved with these new procedures is currently evaluating its own experience. The need for laparoscopic hysterectomy may well vary according to the individual gynaecologist's practice. Those who routinely perform the majority of their hysterectomies by the vaginal route may perhaps find fewer indications than those who usually employ the abdominal technique. There is general agreement that a major advantage of the technique is to transform an abdominal hysterectomy into a vaginal one. Using a combination of operative laparoscopic techniques and vaginal surgery, many patients with endometriosis, pelvic adhesive disease, adnexal disease or benign uterine masses and those who have had previous pelvic surgery can avoid abdominal hysterectomy.

With either traditional abdominal or vaginal hysterectomy, side-wall, pelvic floor, bowel and bladder implants of endometriosis are often missed or remain untreated. Laparoscopic inspection of the pelvis gives a clear magnified view of such implants and with laser or electro-surgical techniques they may be completely removed prior to the hysterectomy. Ovarian endometriomata can also be mobilized and then easily removed vaginally with this technique. Cul-de-sac or stage 4 endometriosis is notoriously difficult to treat at open hysterectomy and is an absolute contraindication to performing vaginal hysterectomy. With care and skill, this most difficult of gynaecological conditions to treat may be effectively managed with a laparoscopic approach (as shown in the series of Figs 5.33–5.63).

The known presence of, or suspicion of, pelvic adhesions is another common indication for choosing to perform an abdominal hysterectomy. Fear of injuring bowel and bladder which may be contained in these adhesions prevents many gynaecologists from removing the uterus vaginally in such cases. With initial diagnostic laparoscopy, the precise extent of the adhesive disease can be determined and, in most cases, with preliminary laparoscopic adhesiolysis, the uterus can be mobilized and safely removed vaginally. Patients who have had previous caesarean sections often have adhesions involving the anterior cul-de-sac, lower uterine segment and bladder. The possible presence of such adhesions is considered by some to be another contraindication to vaginal hyster-ectomy. If such adhesions are present, they can be dissected from the lower segment with laparoscopic scissors or laser and the bladder mobilized from the anterior uterine wall. Following these steps, a vaginal hysterectomy can safely be performed.

Adnexal pathology is usually a contraindication to vaginal hysterectomy. Often the suspected pathology is not present or is found to be a mass of periadnexal adhesions which can be divided laparoscopically prior to a vaginal hysterectomy. If ovarian pathology is present and preliminary ultrasound and CEA 125 estimations combined with the laparoscopic appearance suggest the tumour is benign, then the tumour may be mobilized and, if not grossly enlarged, removed vaginally in a manner similar to that achieved abdominally.

Large uterine myomata are almost invariably removed abdominally. Preliminary endoscopic occlusion of the ovarian and uterine vessels will allow even a large myoma to be morcellated without haemorrhage and the uterus can then be removed vaginally.

Endometrial adenocarcinoma typically occurs in obese, high-risk women. It is important to remove a substantial cuff of vagina and this can perhaps best be done in women of this build with initial laparoscopic inspection and occlusion of the infundibulopelvic and upper uterine vessels laparoscopically, followed by vaginal removal of the uterus with a substantial vaginal cuff produced under direct vision.

In some hands the most frequent indication for laparoscopic hysterectomy will be lack of uterine descent. A well-supported uterus in a nulliparous woman, or one who has had pregnancies delivered abdominally may be difficult to remove vaginally. Such women provide a common and relatively easy indication for laparoscopic hysterectomy. If the surgeon could confidently perform a vaginal hysterectomy in such a case, the vaginal method should remain the preferred method. Laparoscopic hysterectomy, with its greater operating time and operating room costs, should only be performed as an alternative to abdominal and not to vaginal hysterectomy. There will, however, be many indications, for 75% of all hysterectomies are currently performed abdominally.

Recommendations

The precise indications for laparoscopic hysterectomy and laparoscopic-assisted vaginal hysterectomy are not yet clear. Replacing abdominal hysterectomy, however, appears to be the most persuasive reason for attempting this novel, less invasive approach. More accurate haemostasis and lower incidence of haematoma, blood transfusion and postoperative infection are other potential advantages of this approach, as is reduced recovery time.

Laparoscopic hysterectomy: the procedure

Patient position

All prolonged laparoscopic procedures should be performed under general anaesthesia with endotracheal intubation. The routine use of an orogastric tube is recommended to diminish the possibility of a trocar injury to the stomach and to reduce small-bowel distension. The patient is placed flat on the table until the pneumatoperitoneum and the umbilical trocar is inserted. The legs are placed in a 'low' lithotomy position with the hips extended and the thighs supported in a position parallel to the abdomen. Allen stirrups or knee braces or supports which are adjustable to each individual patient are recommended (Fig. 5.7).

The abdominal and vulval skin are cleansed and prepared and the patient is draped. A pelvic examination is performed and, if the patient has not voided immediately before surgery, the bladder is emptied. To give early warning of bladder damage, 15 ml of indigo carmine may be instilled into the bladder at this time. After sounding the uterus, an appropriate size of uterine mobilizer is inserted. A Valtchev uterine mobilizer (Conkin Surgical Instruments, Toronto, Ont.) is recommended because it gives a secure hold and considerable mobility (see Fig. 4.1). Four interchangeable, detachable, uterine obturators range in length from 4.5 to 10 cm and from 3 to 10 mm in thickness (see Fig. 4.2). With a 10 mm × 10 cm obturator fixed into position, the uterus can be flexed through 120° and can be moved in an arc of 45° to the right or left (Fig. 5.8).

When the umbilical trocar is *in situ*, the patient is placed in a steep Trendelenberg position. If a tilt of 30° or more can be obtained, the view deep into the pelvis will be improved and such an angle is recommended (Fig. 5.9). Few modern operating tables can give such a steep degree of tilt. The hand-operated Champagne model 600 (Affiliated Table Company, Rochester, NY) can be used in conjunction with supportive shoulder braces.

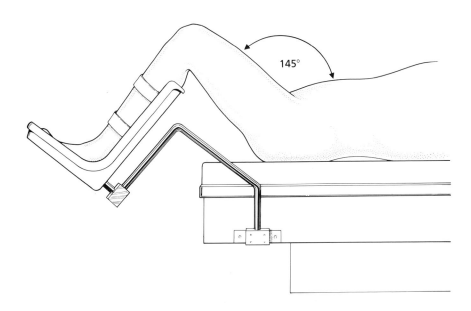

Fig. 5.7 Optimum patient position for laparoscopic hysterectomy.

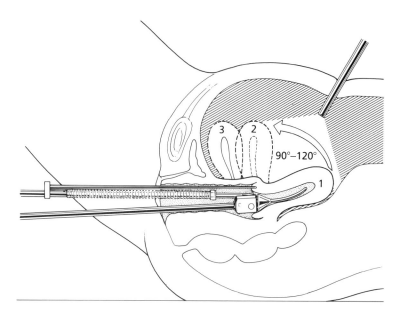

Fig. 5.8 Diagram demonstrating mobility of uterus with Valtchev's manipulator *in situ*.

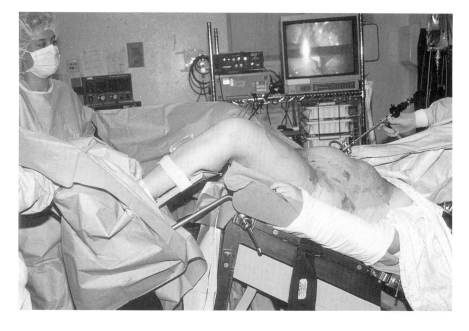

Fig. 5.9 Patient in 30° Trendelenberg position.

Positioning of the equipment

A great deal of special equipment is required during any advanced laparoscopic procedure and it is important that all this equipment is conveniently located. It is preferable to group it in tower stacks with complementary items arranged together. The gynaecologist stands on the patient's left and a specially trained assistant stands between the patient's legs (Figs 5.10 and 5.11). If available, a second assistant can stand on the patient's right side. The first video-monitor is on the top shelf of a stack placed on the patient's right side level with her hip. This should be angled to give the operator an optimum view. Below this should be placed the light source and the video-camera control

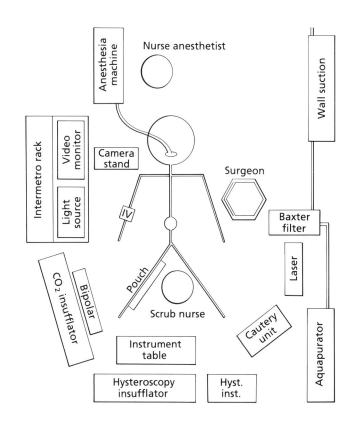

Fig. 5.10 Reich's recommended positioning of equipment around patient.

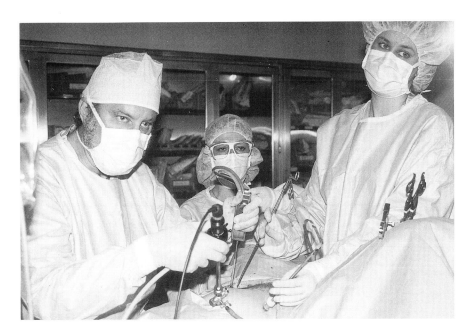

Fig. 5.11 Position of surgeon and second nurse on patient's left with first assistant standing between the patient's legs.

unit and video recording apparatus (see Fig. 3.5). If a second monitor is available, it should be placed behind the gynaecologist and again placed on the top shelf of a stack and angled so that both assistants can see it. Beneath this monitor can be placed the electronic CO_2 insufflator and the aquadissection apparatus (see Fig. 4.19).

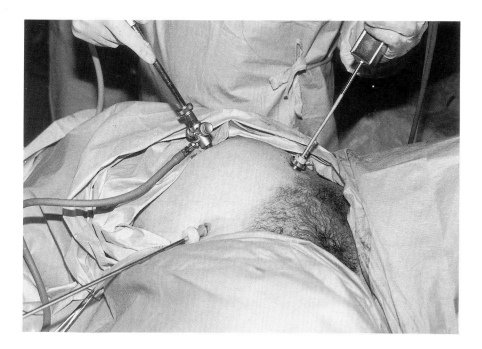

Fig. 5.12 Reich's working set up for laparoscopic hysterectomy with one 10-mm portal in the umbilicus and two 5-mm portals in the lower abdomen.

The abdominal incisions

Three or four laparoscopic puncture sites are used. Reich always uses a three-portal approach with a vertical intraumbilical incision, made to accommodate a 10-mm laparoscope (see Fig. 4.9). Two lower-quadrant pubic hair-line incisions to accommodate 5-mm trocars are also made (see Figs 4.13 and 4.14). These are placed laterally to the inferior epigastric vessels and the rectus abdominis muscle as described in Chapter 4 (Fig. 5.12). Other workers describe a third, lower incision. If used, this is placed in the midline above the pubic hair-line, usually at a higher level than the two lateral portals. This third portal will be either 5 or 12 mm in size; the larger size will be chosen if Endo GIA staples are to be applied. C.Y. Liu uses a 12-mm umbilical and four 5-mm secondary punctures, two placed low in the left and right iliac fossae and two higher in the same vertical line, inserted just below the level of the umbilicus. Garry recommends three secondary-puncture portals. Two are placed in the low-lateral positions previously described and the third at the level of, and to the left of, the umbilical incision (Figs 5.13–5.15). This configuration is preferred because it allows the Endo GIA stapling device and the bipolar diathermy forceps to be introduced parallel to and close to the uterus, in a similar manner to that achieved during a standard abdominal hysterectomy.

The pneumatoperitoneum

The pneumatoperitoneum is induced after inserting a sharp Veress needle through the intraumbilical incision. This is connected to a high-

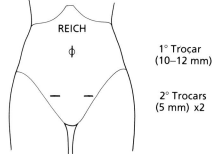

Fig. 5.13 Reich's recommended portals of entry.

Fig. 5.14 Liu's suggested portals of entry.

Fig. 5.15 Garry's modifications to the recommended points of entry for laparoscopic hysterectomy.

inflow electronic insufflator and CO_2 is used to distend the cavity. Once a free flow is established, gas is instilled at the rate of 3−4 litres/min until adequate abdominal distension is produced. The operating pressure should be preset and controlled between 10 and 15 mmHg but some operators prefer to temporarily increase the abdominal pressure to 25 mmHg during the initial insertion of the trocars. This higher pressure produces an abdominal wall under tension, through which it is easier to insert the trocars.

Preliminary inspection

The abdominal cavity, particularly the pelvis, is carefully inspected and the nature and extent of any pathology carefully documented. Abdominal and adnexal adhesions, if present, are divided with scissors and diathermy or lasers.

Operative technique

Reich describes a six-stage technique for TLH.

Stage 1: Demonstration of the ureters

The ureters should always be clearly identified at the pelvic brim and may be dissected to clearly demonstrate their course. Most American authorities agree with Reich, who suggests that such a formal dissection of the ureter is an essential first step in this procedure which should be done in every case. He recommends that this is done first before the pelvic side-wall peritoneum becomes oedematous and/or opaque from irritation by the CO_2 pneumatoperitoneum or aquadissection and before ureteral peristalsis is inhibited by surgical stress, pressure or the Trendelenberg position. Many European authorities, including the Clermont-Ferrand school argue that this is not usually done at the time of open abdominal hysterectomy and, if performed with careful technique, should not be necessary in many laparoscopic hysterectomies either. All authorities agree that, whether the ureters are formally dissected out or not, it is essential that their location is determined and all operative procedures are performed well clear of them. If there is pathology high on the pelvic side-wall or in the ovarian fossa, ureteric dissection should begin at the pelvic brim. This is usually easy on the right side, where the ureter is readily visualized, but it is often more difficult on the left side, where the course of the ureter is often covered by the rectosigmoid colon. This should be first freed and reflected from the left iliac fossa to expose the ovarian vessels, the ureter, and the superior rectal vessels as they cross over the iliac artery and enter the true pelvis (Fig. 5.16). The ureter may be formally dissected at the pelvic brim level but this is usually only necessary when it cannot

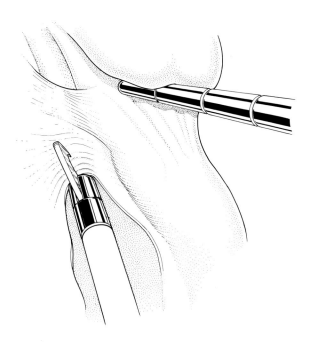

Fig. 5.16 Initial incision with scissors into pelvic side-wall peritoneum to allow demonstration of the ureter.

easily be seen through the peritoneum. In the absence of upper pelvic side-wall pathology, it is better to trace the course of the ureter down the pelvic side-wall and grasp it low in the pelvis, just above its entrance to the ureteric canal. An atraumatic grasping forceps is used from a right-sided cannula to grab the ureter and its overlying peritoneum on the left pelvic side-wall below and caudad to the left ovary, lateral to the left uterosacral ligament. Scissors can be used to divide the peritoneum overlying the ureter and are then inserted into the defect and spread. Thereafter, one blade of the scissors is placed on top of the ureter, the buried scissor blade visualized through the peritoneum and the peritoneum divided. This is continued into the deep pelvis where the uterine vessels cross the ureter. Connective tissue between the ureter and the vessels is divided with sharp-scissors dissection and any bleeding is controlled with well-insulated bipolar forceps. This dissection can alternatively be performed with CO_2 laser or with Nd-YAG laser and sapphire scalpel tip (Fig. 5.17a−c).

Stage 2: Bladder mobilization

The left round ligament is divided at its mid-portion with either a spoon electrode at 150W cutting current or bipolar coagulation and scissors or Nd-YAG laser with scalpel tip (Fig. 5.18). Persistent bleeding is controlled, either with unipolar fulguration at 80W coagulation current or bipolar desiccation at 30W cutting current. Scissors are then used to divide the vesicouterine peritoneal fold, starting at the left side and continuing across the midline to the right round ligament (Figs 5.19 and 5.20). The right round ligament is then divided in a similar manner.

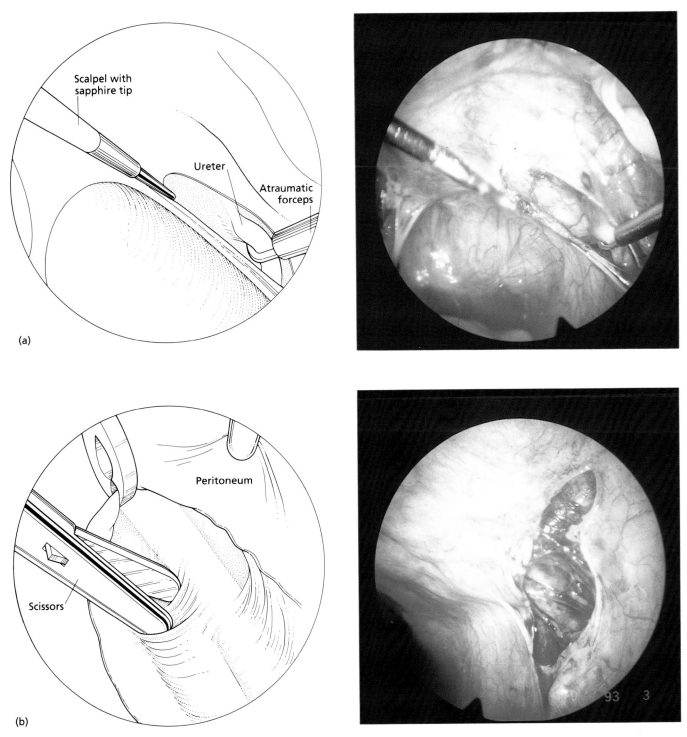

Fig. 5.17 (a) The ureter being dissected. This can be done with scissors, CO_2 laser or as here with Nd-YAG laser. (b) The dissection being extended with scissors, grasping forceps and aquadissection.

(*continued overleaf*)

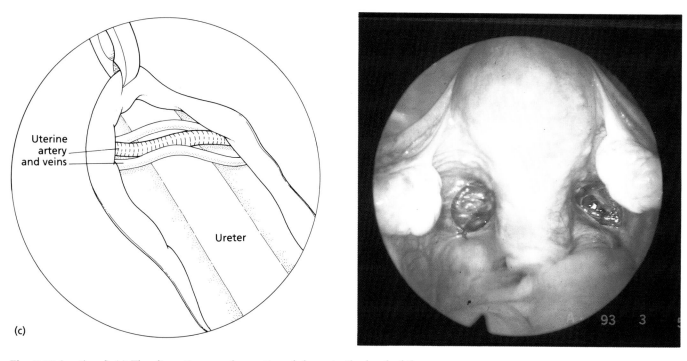

Fig. 5.17 (*continued*) (c) The dissection may be continued down to the level of the uterine vessels.

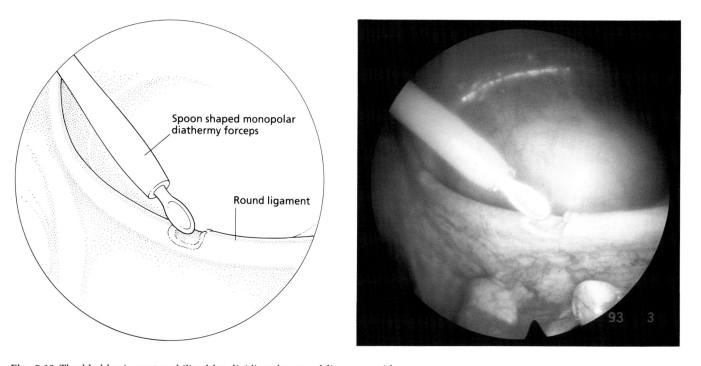

Fig. 5.18 The bladder is next mobilized by dividing the round ligament with monopolar diathermy or bipolar diathermy plus cutting with scissors, CO_2 or Nd-YAG laser.

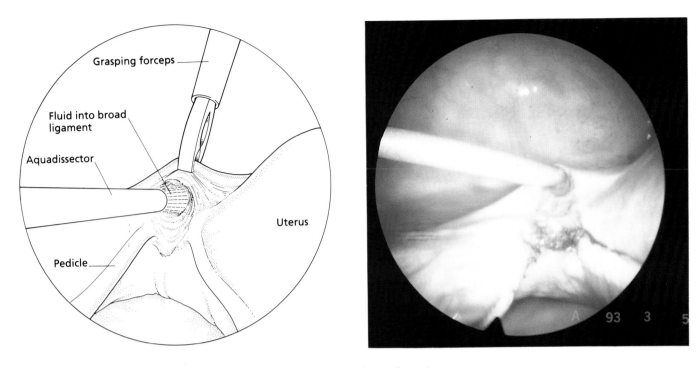

Fig. 5.19 The vesicouterine peritoneum is elevated with forceps and aquadissection.

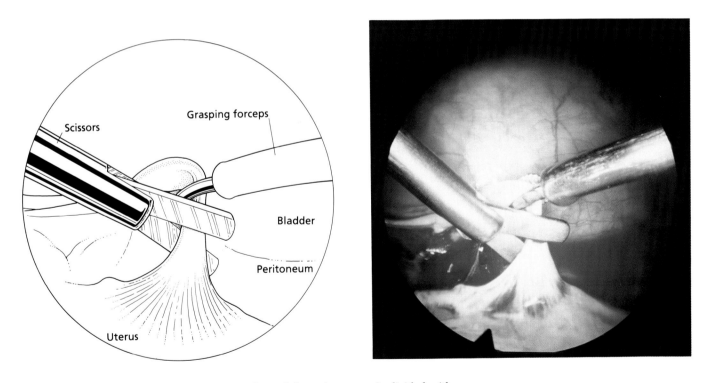

Fig. 5.20 The bladder flap peritoneum once elevated from the uterus is divided with any of the cutting modalities available.

The bladder is then freed from the uterus and upper vagina with scissors.

Stage 3: Upper uterine blood supply

When the ovaries are to be conserved, the most convenient way to divide the upper uterine blood supply is with the Endo GIA. To minimize the number of large trocar incisions the 10-mm telescope is removed from the 12-mm trocar sheath placed in the umbilicus and is replaced by a 5-mm telescope placed in the left lateral port (or the upper left lateral port if Garry's configuration has been selected). The Endo GIA is then inserted through the 12-mm umbilical trocar and applied to the utero-ovarian ligament and fallopian tube near the uterus (Fig. 5.21). When the position has been carefully checked, the stapling instrument is fired and, when the jaws are opened, the staple line is carefully checked for bleeding and completeness of tissue division (Fig. 5.22). If the ovaries are to be removed, there is less advantage in using the Endo GIA and the infundibulopelvic ligament and its contained vessels can be divided by taking a series of small bites with the bipolar forceps and desiccating the tissue (Fig. 5.23a—d). This can then be divided with scissors or Nd-YAG laser and the relatively bloodless line of dissection can be progressively advanced by alternating desiccation and cutting until the broad ligaments are opened.

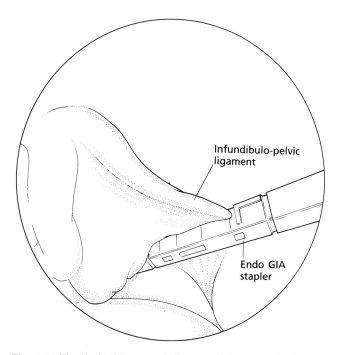 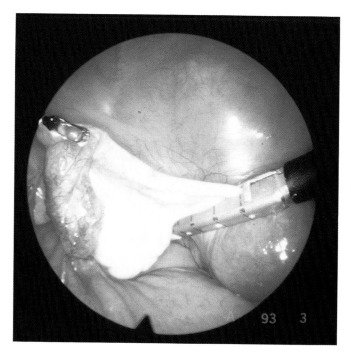

Fig. 5.21 The Endo GIA' 30 multifine staple being applied to the left round ligament and infundibulopelvic ligaments simultaneously.

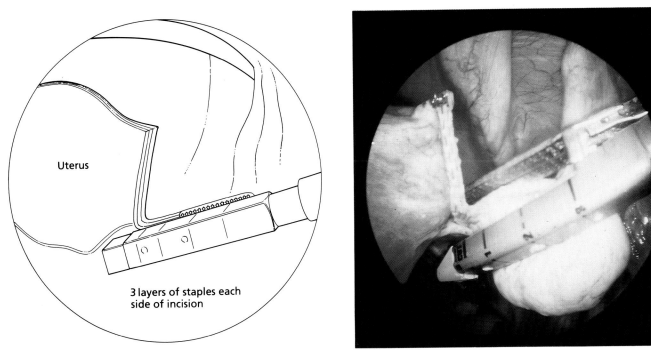

Fig. 5.22 The triple layer of staples left either side of the 3-cm long incision should be inspected for completeness of haemostasis.

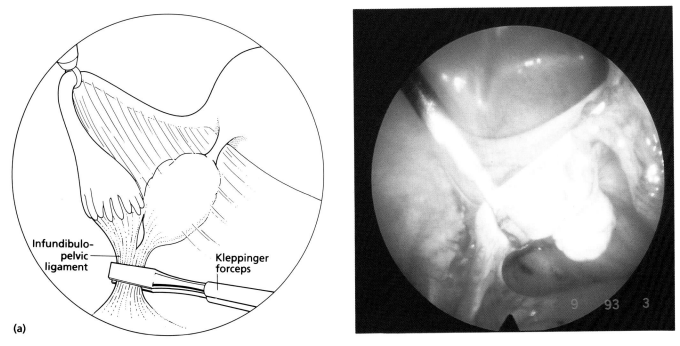

Fig. 5.23 (a) The left infundibulo-pelvic ligament is secured by taking a series of bites with the Kleppinger forceps and coagulating small segments of tissue.

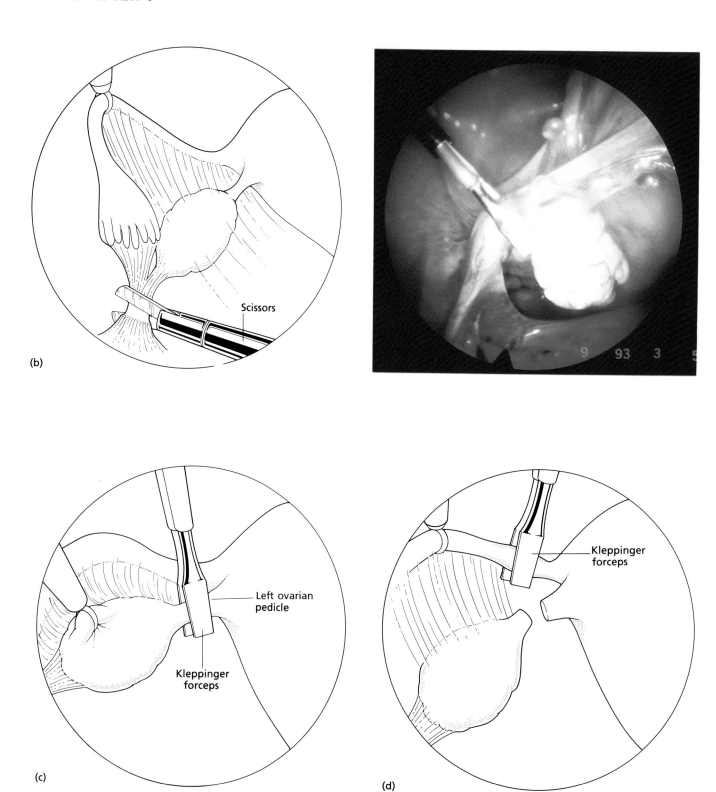

(b)

(c)

(d)

Scissors

Left ovarian
pedicle

Kleppinger
forceps

Kleppinger
forceps

Fig. 5.23 (*continued*) (b) The desiccated tissue is then divided with scissors or laser and the procedure repeated until all the tissue is divided without blood loss. (c, d) This technique can also be used if the ovaries are to be conserved and will be effective providing appropriately small bites are taken. Here the ovarian ligament is secured. (c) The left ovarian pedicle is desiccated. (d) The left ovarian ligament is further desiccated.

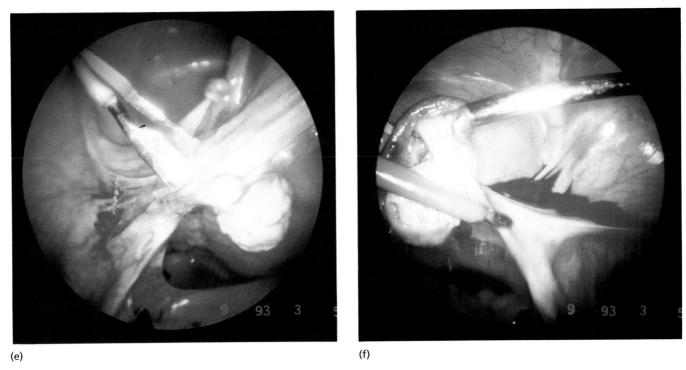

(e)

(f)

Fig. 5.23 (*continued*) (e) The left infundibulopelvic ligament is desiccated. The left fallopian tube is desiccated with the bipolar forceps. (f) The desiccated ligament is divided with monopolar diathermy.

Stage 4: Uterine-vessel ligation

The broad ligament on each side is skeletonized down to the uterine vessels. Each uterine vessel pedicle is then secured. Reich now recommends that this should be done by suture ligation with o Vicryl on a CT 1 needle or o Polysorb on a GS 21 needle. The needles are introduced down the lower left 5-mm trocar incision (Fig. 5.24). The curved needle is inserted on top of the unroofed ureter where it turns medially towards the previously mobilized bladder (Fig. 5.25). A short rotary movement of the Cook oblique-curved needle-holder brings the needle around the uterine-vessel pedicle. Sutures are tied extracorporeally, using a Clarke knot-pusher. A single suture placed in this manner acts as a 'sentinel stitch' identifying the artery and protecting the ureter for the rest of the case. The uterine artery may also be secured with bipolar diathermy coagulation, the application of single clips or the application of a further Endo GIA staple cartridge. If these techniques are used it is essential to visualize the ureter and to determine its relation to the artery.

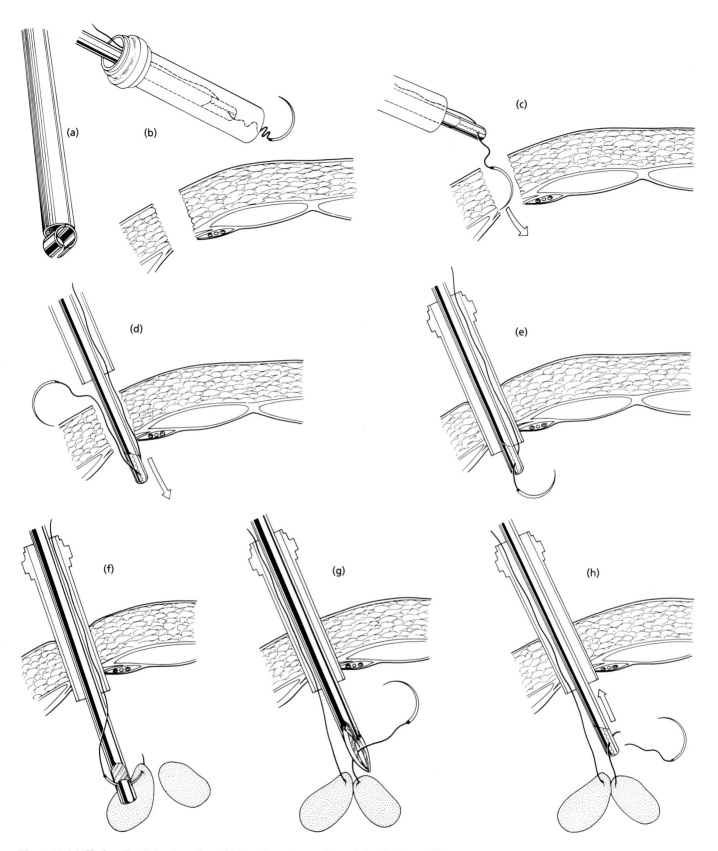

Fig. 5.24 (a) Clarke–Reich knot-pusher. (b) The short trocar sleeve is loaded by pulling the suture material up the barrel from the distal to the proximal end of the shaft. (c) The needle-holder is then reintroduced down the sheath and closed around the suture just behind the swarf of the needle. (d) The needle-holder is then reintroduced into the abdominal cavity pulling the needle after it. (e) Inside the cavity the needle is released and then regrasped in the standard manner. (f) The needle is driven through the tissues to be ligated. (g) The needle and 3 cm of suture are then divided and the needle is safely parked in the peritoneum. (h) The suture is regrasped and pulled back up through the trocar sleeve.

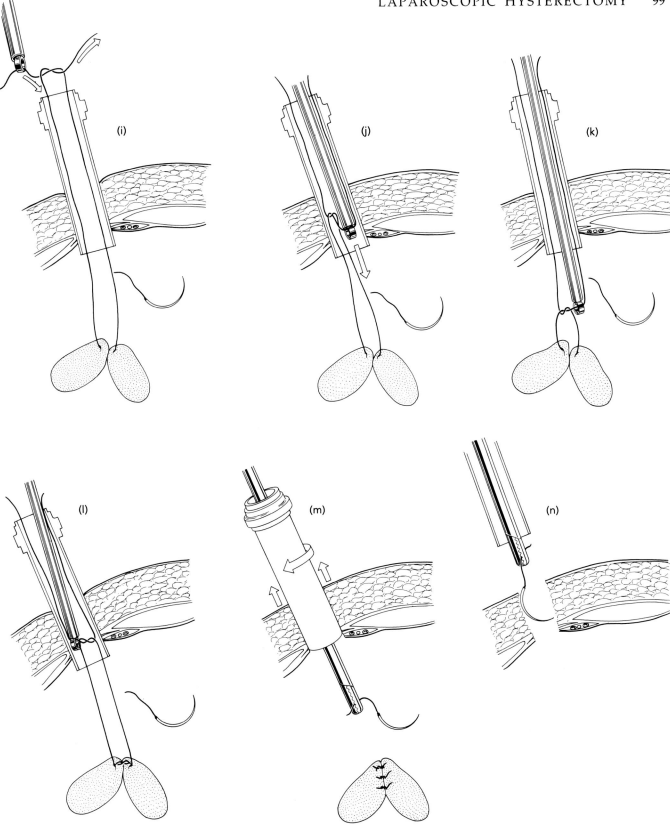

Fig. 5.24 (*continued*) (i) A single throw hitch is formed. (j) The throw is pushed down into the abdomen with the knot-pusher. (k) The knot is tightened on the tissue. (l) A second throw is formed and this is also pushed down into the abdomen. (m) When the suture is tied and the ends cut, the suture attached to the needle is grasped and pulled into the abdominal wall. (n) The trocar with suture and needle are then removed from the abdomen as one. The trocar sheath is then reinserted into the stab incision. Reproduced with permission from The American College of Obstetricians and Gynecologists (*Obstetrics and Gynecology* 1992; **79**: 143–147).

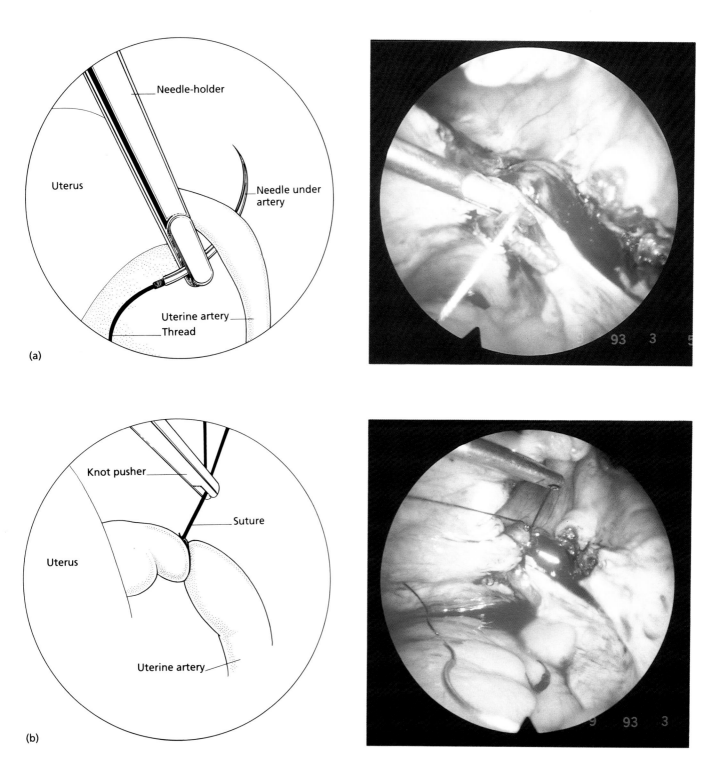

Fig. 5.25 (a) The uterine artery can be ligated with a curved needle inserted above the ureter and below the artery. (b) The artery is then ligated twice.

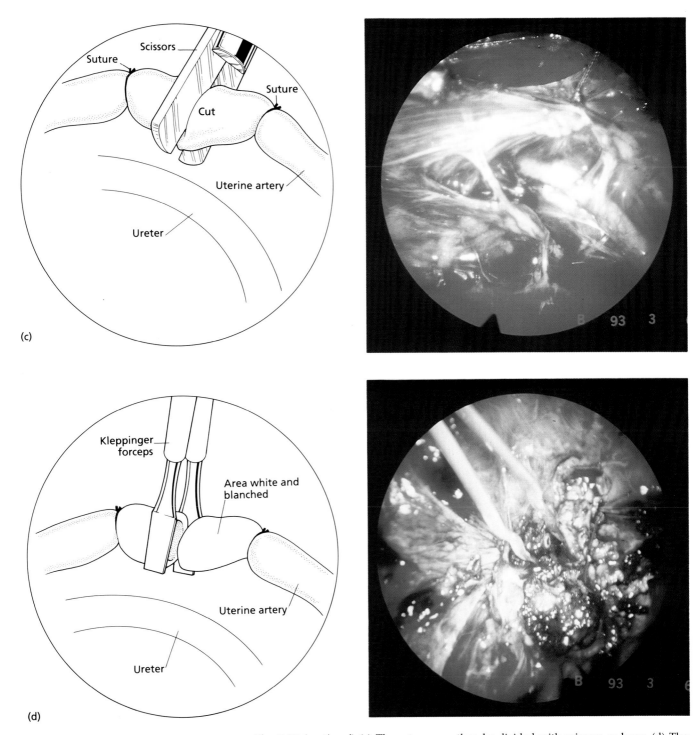

Fig. 5.25 (*continued*) (c) The artery may then be divided with scissors or laser. (d) The cut ends must be carefully inspected to ensure adequate haemostasis.

Stage 5: Circumferential culdotomy (division of the cervicovaginal attachments)

The cardinal ligaments are best divided with the CO_2 laser at high power (80 W) or the spoon electrode at 150 W. Bleeding will require control with bipolar diathermy. The vagina is entered posteriorly (Fig. 5.26) over the Valtchev retractor, which identifies the junction of the cervix with the vagina. The rectum can be identified by manipulation of a probe.

Continuing towards the left side, the anterior vaginal fornix is divided. The suction–irrigation probe can then be inserted into the incision and is then used as a backstop and the anterior fornix is also divided. The anterior fornix is tented by an assistant moving a ring forceps in the fornix (Fig. 5.27). This tenting allows precise dissection of the bladder off the anterior vaginal wall. The probe is inserted from posterior to anterior to delineate the right vagina. The uterus is then pulled out of the vagina (Fig. 5.28). During these latter manoeuvres, a swab in a condom is placed in the vagina to help maintain the pneumatoperitoneum. When the uterus is pulled into the vagina the swab is removed and replaced with the fundus of the uterus which acts as an effective 'cork' for the vagina and maintains the pneumatoperitoneum (Fig. 5.29).

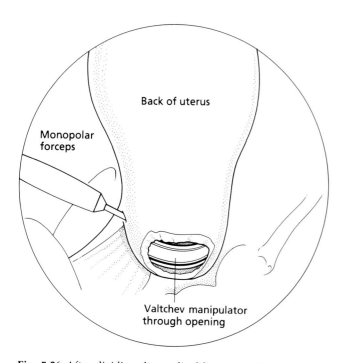

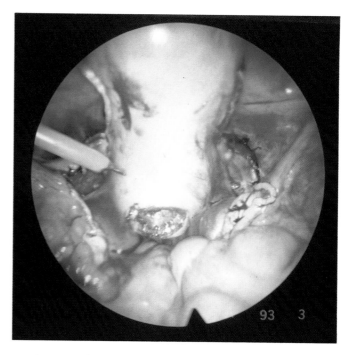

Fig. 5.26 After dividing the cardinal ligaments the vagina may be entered posteriorly using monopolar diathermy or laser. Care is taken to ensure the rectum has been reflected and the vagina is entered over the Valtchev retractor.

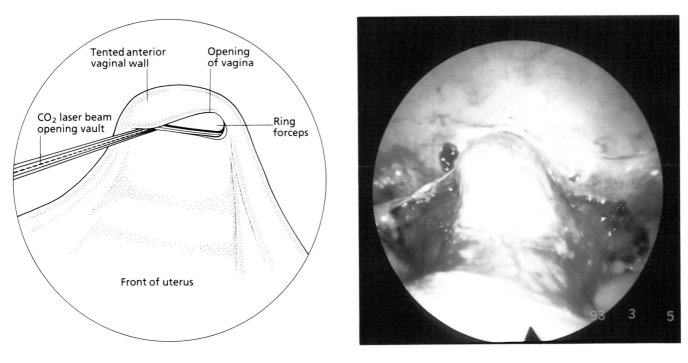

Fig. 5.27 The anterior vaginal fornix may be entered by tenting it with a ring forceps placed in the vagina by an assistant.

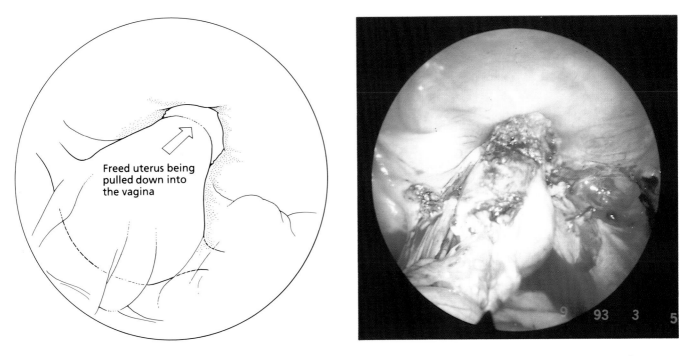

Fig. 5.28 The freed uterus is then pulled out of the abdomen through the colpotomy incision.

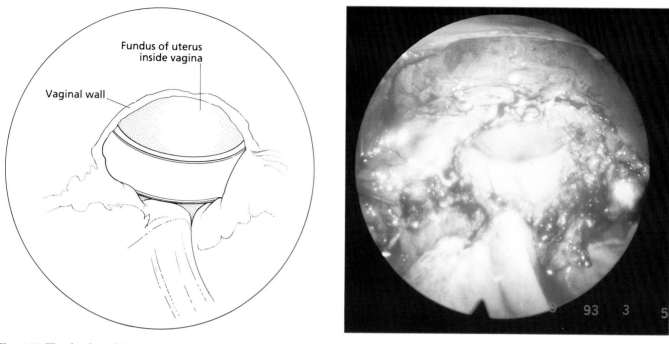

Fig. 5.29 The fundus of the uterus is left in the upper vagina to act as a 'plug' and prevent the loss of the pneumatoperitoneum.

Stage 6: Laparoscopic vaginal vault closure with McCall culdoplasty

The left uterosacral ligament and posterolateral vagina are first elevated. A suture is placed through this uterosacral ligament and into the vagina, and then it exits the vagina again to include the posterior

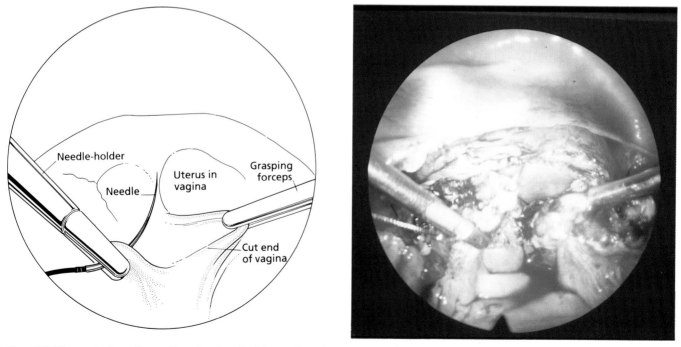

Fig. 5.30 The vaginal vault may then be closed with a series of extracorporeal tied laparoscopic sutures. The vault may be supported by performing a McCall culdoplasty.

vaginal tissue near the midline on the left and re-enters just adjacent to this spot on the right. Finally, an opposite-side oblique Cook needle-holder is used to fixate the right posterolateral vagina to the right uterosacral ligament. This suture is tied extracorporeally and gives excellent support to the vaginal cuff apex, elevating it superiorly and back towards the hollow of the sacrum. The rest of the vagina and overlying pubocervical fascia are closed vertically with a figure-of-eight suture (Fig. 5.30).

Posthysterectomy laparoscopic inspection

After closing the vaginal vault, the abdomen is reinflated and the operative sites are again carefully inspected laparoscopically. Blood clots are identified and aspirated (Fig. 5.31). All pedicles are carefully inspected for bleeding. Haemostasis is achieved with bipolar compression and desiccation (Fig. 5.32), ligation with clips or staples or coagulation with an argon-beam coagulator.

With a standard pneumatoperitoneum, the CO_2 is maintained at a pressure of 10–15 mmHg and this may effectively tamponade some opened small vessels, which may bleed again once the tamponade effect is released. Complete haemostasis can therefore be better confirmed by replacing the CO_2 with several litres of Ringer's lactate or normal saline and then performing an underwater inspection of the operative sites. The patient's position may be altered from Trendelenberg to flat to reverse Trendelenberg to ensure adequate visualization.

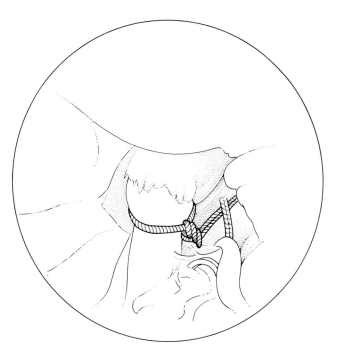

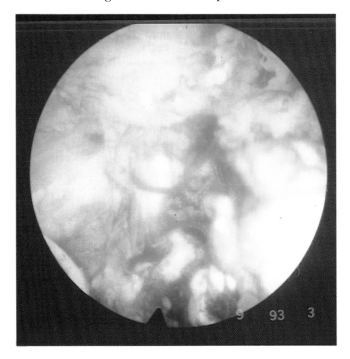

Fig. 5.31 On completion of the procedure the pelvis is filled with sodium chloride or Ringer's lactate and all suture lines are inspected under water to ensure complete haemostasis.

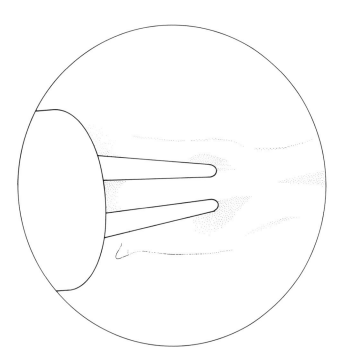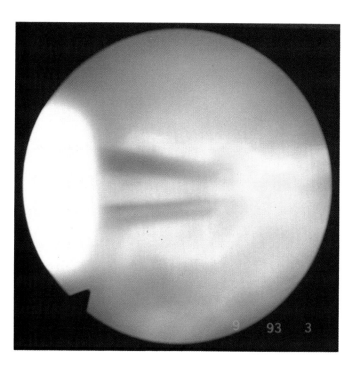

Fig. 5.32 Additional haemostasis produced under water with the micro bipolar forceps.

Haemostasis is then achieved with bipolar compression and desiccation. This liberal irrigation removes any blood clot and debris from the abdominal cavity. This may also reduce any possible focus for subsequent infection and 1–2 litres of irrigating fluid are left in the cavity at the end of the procedure.

Completion of the procedure

All the secondary trocars are removed under continued laparoscopic inspection and the abdominal incisions closed. Simple approximation is adequate for incisions of 5 mm or less but for those larger than this the deep fascia should be identified and separately approximated to reduce the risk of subsequent incisional herniation.

The above text has described the stages required to perform a total laparoscopic hysterectomy and such procedures have been performed many times now by numerous different gynaecologists. The fact that such a procedure is technically possible is not, however, an indication to perform it. Such techniques demand a high level of competence at advanced laparoscopic surgery, much expensive and novel equipment and, above all, considerable time and commitment. The most difficult stage of the operation technically is the control of the uterine vessels and the identification of the ureter at the level of the ureteric canal. Mobilization of the adnexal structures, securing the infundibulopelvic ligaments and reflecting the bladder from the anterior surface of the uterus are relatively straightforward laparoscopic procedures. These steps are, however, the most difficult stages in a standard vaginal hysterectomy. Clamping the uterosacral and cardinal ligaments and controlling the uterine vessels are the simplest stages in a vaginal hysterectomy.

The principal objective of laparoscopic assistance during hysterectomy is to avoid the need for an abdominal wall scar and the morbidity associated with large skin incisions. A consensus is evolving among laparoscopic surgeons that, in each individual patient, a decision must be taken as to how much of the hysterectomy should be done laparoscopically and how much vaginally. As, in general terms, the vaginal portion of the operation is usually quicker and uses cheaper materials and equipment, the principle should be to only do laparoscopically those stages which cannot easily be done vaginally. In most cases, this will involve laparoscopically dividing any pelvic adhesions and ablating any endometriotic implants, mobilizing the adnexa, securing the infundibulopelvic vessels and possibly reflecting the bladder from the uterus. The remainder of the procedure can be completed vaginally before returning for a final laparoscopic inspection and abdominal irrigation.

Many cases of laparoscopic hysterectomy will be done with difficult pathology. In such cases it is essential that the ureters are dissected out. Figures 5.33–5.63 clearly demonstrate the procedure in such a difficult case.

Vaginal procedures

The CO_2 insufflation is discontinued but the laparoscopic instruments are left in the operating portals. The patient should be repositioned in the surgeon's standard manner for a vaginal hysterectomy. It is important to have maximum access at this time and a higher lithotomy position is usually preferred.

A speculum or a retractor is placed in the posterior fornix and a Wertheim's or Heaney retractor is placed in the anterior fornix to hold the bladder away from the cervix. The cervix is held with vulsellum forceps and a circular incision made with a scalpel. The anterior fornix is entered and, if the bladder has been previously reflected, this is usually extremely easy. A suction catheter should be available to remove any residual irrigation fluid, which will rapidly drain. The pouch of Douglas is also opened and the undivided cardinal and uterosacral ligaments clamped and secured with sutures in the standard manner. If the uterine vessels have not previously been secured laparoscopically, they can at this stage be clamped and tied vaginally. The completely mobilized uterus, with or without the ovaries and tubes, can then be delivered vaginally.

The peritoneum can be closed, the uterosacral ligaments approximated and the vaginal skin closed transversely with a series of interrup-

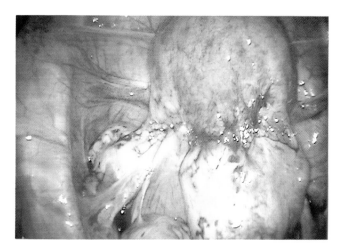

Fig. 5.33 Pelvis before surgery with severe stage 4 endometriosis and bilateral endometriomata and complete cul-de-sac obliteration.

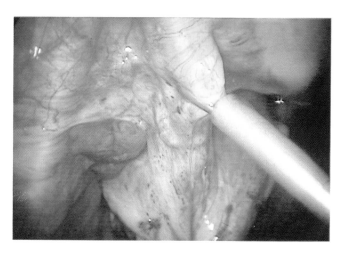

Fig. 5.36 The pelvic peritoneum is grasped and the course of the ureter defined.

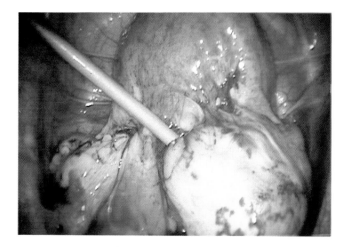

Fig. 5.34 First the endometriomata are drained.

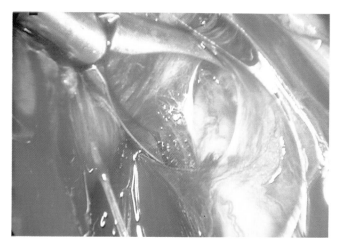

Fig. 5.37 The peritoneum is opened and the ureter displayed.

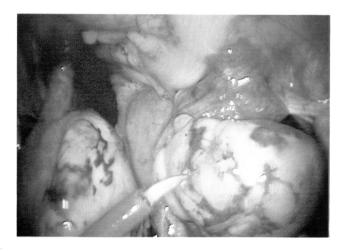

Fig. 5.35 The uterus and adnexal structures are then mobilized.

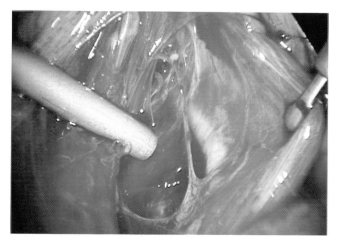

Fig. 5.38 With aquadissection, and sharp and blunt conventional dissection the ureter is more completely visualized.

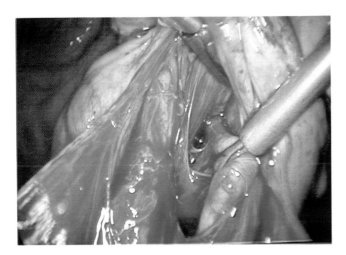

Fig. 5.39 It is possible to pick up the ureter with atraumatic forceps.

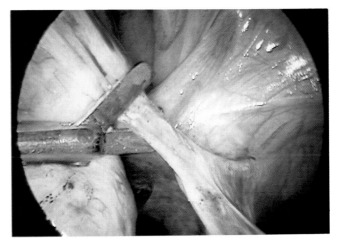

Fig. 5.42 After desiccation the infundibulopelvic ligament is divided with scissors (CO_2 or Nd-YAG laser or monopolar diathermy can also be used).

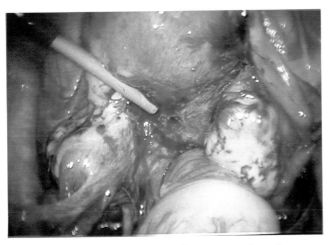

Fig. 5.40 When the procedure has been repeated on the opposite side and both ureters have been clearly defined and the uterus and adnexa are mobile, the total laparoscopic hysterectomy is begun.

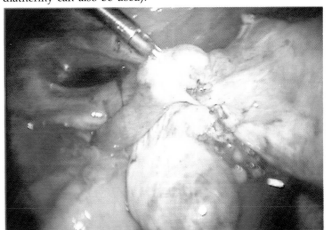

Fig. 5.43 The dissection is continued by taking a series of small bites with the bipolar forceps and after desiccation dividing the tissue.

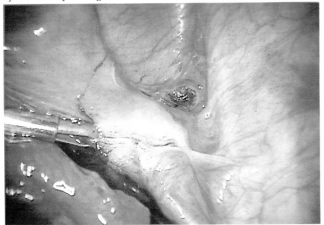

Fig. 5.41 The round ligaments are grasped with Kleppinger bipolar forceps and the tissue desiccated.

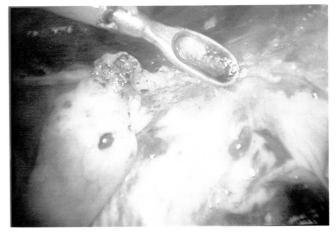

Fig. 5.44 The tissue is again divided with monopolar electrode scissors or laser. The procedure is repeated — desiccation, division, desiccation, division — until the uterine arteries are displayed.

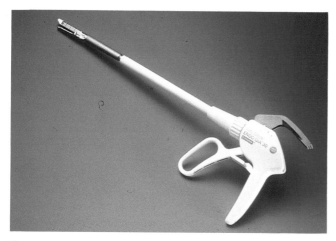

Fig. 5.45 Alternatively these pedicles can be secured with the AutoSuture Multifine Endo GIA 30.

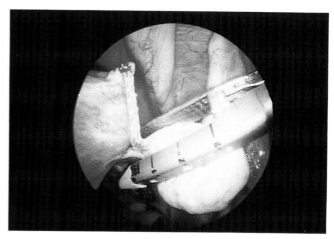

Fig. 5.48 On reopening the jaws the tissues separate.

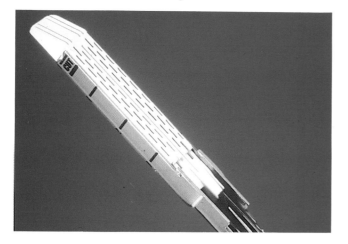

Fig. 5.46 The Endo GIA fires six rows of titanium staples and automatically divides between them leaving two pedicles with three rows of staples on each side.

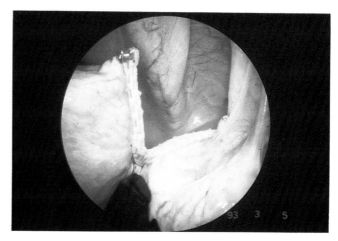

Fig. 5.49 Three rows of staples on each side of the pedicle can be seen.

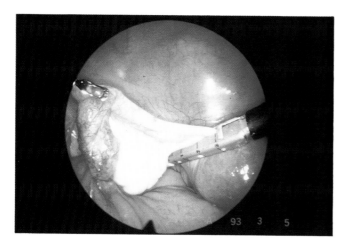

Fig. 5.47 The jaws of the Endo GIA are opened and placed over the pedicle to be secured. The jaws are then closed and the handles squeezed to fire the staple.

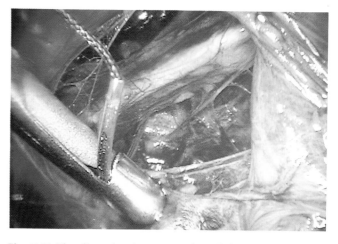

Fig. 5.50 The dissection is continued until the uterine arteries are demonstrated. They are then secured by suturing. The curved needle is inserted above the ureter and under the uterine artery.

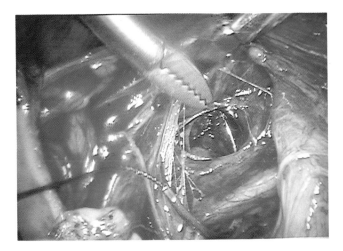

Fig. 5.51 The needle is drawn around the artery.

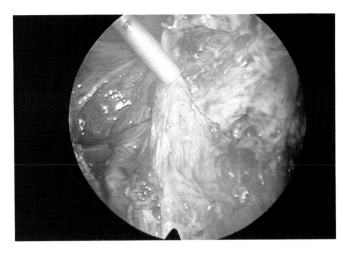

Fig. 5.54 The uterus is then further mobilized. Endometriotic tissue is removed from the cul-de-sac and the rectum reflected away from the posterior fornix.

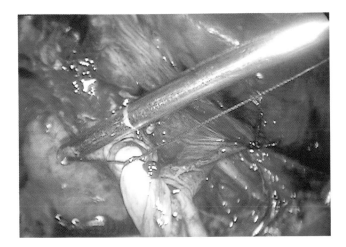

Fig. 5.52 An extracorporeal hitch is formed and pushed firmly down onto the vessel with a Clarke−Reich knot-pusher.

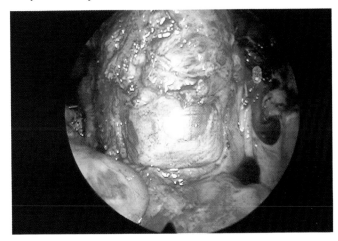

Fig. 5.55 The posterior cul-de-sac is open with high-powered CO_2 laser monopolar diathermy or scissors.

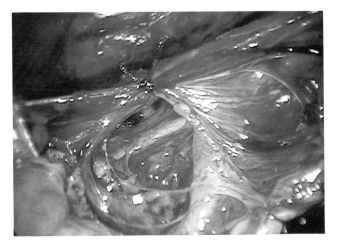

Fig. 5.53 The ends of the sutures are divided and the procedure repeated and the artery divided on both sides.

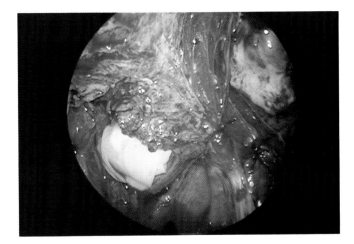

Fig. 5.56 The excision is extended laterally and haemostasis secured.

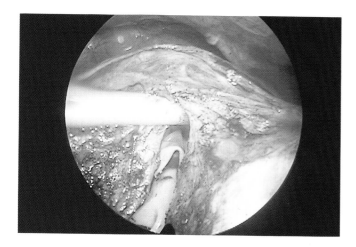

Fig. 5.57 The anterior fornix is tented and opened in a similar manner.

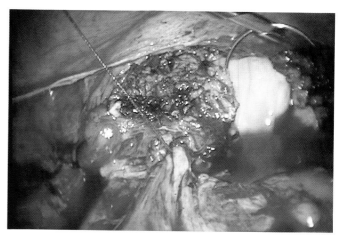

Fig. 5.60 The vaginal vault is closed with a series of sutures applied laparoscopically.

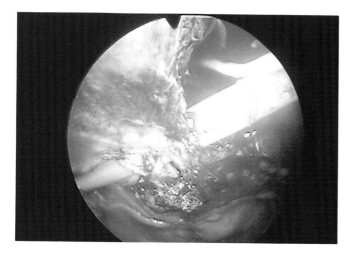

Fig. 5.58 The two incisions are joined by extending them laterally.

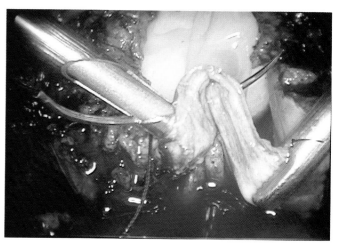

Fig. 5.61 The suture includes the uterosacral and cardinal ligaments and the vaginal mucosa on each side.

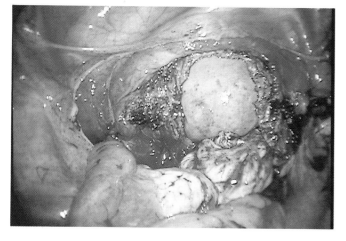

Fig. 5.59 The now completely mobilized uterus is pulled from below down into the vagina.

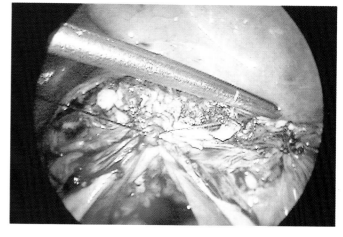

Fig. 5.62 The suture is tied extracorporeally and ligated closing off the vagina.

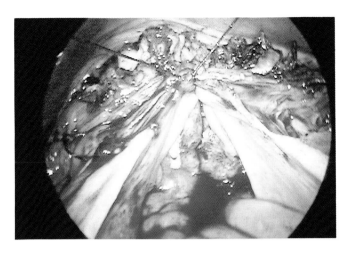

Fig. 5.63 The procedure is repeated until the vault is closed and haemostatic.

ted sutures. When haemostasis is secured the CO_2 insufflation is restarted and the cavity inspected and irrigated as previously described.

Special problems related to laparoscopic hysterectomy

Many difficulties may be encountered during the division of the lateral cervix from the vagina because of ascending vaginal vessels and thick cardinal and uterosacral ligaments. It is difficult to maintain the CO_2 pneumatoperitoneum once the vagina has been opened. To overcome this difficulty, the vagina may be packed but the bulk of the uterine manipulator may prevent an airtight closure being produced. It is often better at this stage to remove the manipulator and tenaculum from the vagina and replace it with a wet pack or a pack inside a surgical glove. The cervix can then be divided from its junction with the vagina by lifting the anterior vaginectomy to put the cervicovaginal junction on tension, and dividing this junction with scissors through 360° until the uterus is free in the peritoneal cavity. Scissors with electrosurgical capability can reduce bleeding from the cuff. The scissors are used to grasp the junction, cutting current is applied, and the cervicovaginal tissue is divided.

After completely freeing the cervix, it is grasped with a tenaculum and the uterus is pulled into the vagina. If it is too large for this manoeuvre, the surgeon can go vaginally to morcellate the uterus. If this is not necessary, the uterus is pulled into the vagina and left in such a position that the fundus occludes the canal and helps maintain the pneumatoperitoneum. The vaginal cuff is carefully inspected for bleeding at this time. Bleeding at this site may be fulgurized with unipolar coagulation current, argon-beam coagulator or bipolar desiccation. The cuff is then closed with three sutures of 0 Vicryl on a CT 1 needle. The first suture approximates the uterosacral ligaments across the midline. The second suture brings together the cardinal ligaments and underlying vagina. The third suture closes the anterior vagina and its pubocervical fascia.

Removal of large masses

For large fibroid hysterectomies, an 11-mm cork-screw is screwed into the myoma vaginally through the culdotomy incision. The myoma is thereby put on traction and further morcellated with scissors or scalpel until removal is complete. Large masses can be removed through small culdotomy incisions in this way. These large masses regularly include 10–15-cm fibroids and ovarian fibroma (the largest weighing 875 g). Even larger fibroids may be removed through the vaginal cuff with morcellation. This can be time-consuming and may require up to an hour of painstaking morcellation to complete. It is wise to change from laparoscopic stirrups (Allen stirrups or knee supports) to candy-cane stirrups to obtain better hip flexion in order to permit assistance with vaginal side-wall retractors during long procedures. Self-retaining lateral vaginal-wall retractors are considered for shorter procedures.

To gain an initial grip on the mass to be delivered an 11-mm laparoscopic cork-screw (Wisap, Tomball, TX) is inserted through the vaginal cuff for a culdotomy incision. A second 11-mm cork-screw is inserted alongside the first one and, using a scalpel, the myoma is divided between the two cork-screw devices. The leading cork-screw with surrounding tissue is incised with a scalpel or scissors so that a wedge of fibroid is freed from the larger body of the mass. An apple-coring technique can be performed with traction around the second cork-screw. The scalpel encircles the myoma to remove a large core. The soft tissue of the uterus will often invert during this procedure to permit delivery of much of the lesion. Myomata, however, seldom lose their shape unless degenerative changes have occurred. Much morcellation is often required but a surgeon's patience and hard work can be rewarded by accomplishing the removal of large-sized masses of over 1000 g.

The procedure for the removal of such very large fibroids is as follows:

1 Establish pneumatoperitoneum through a standard intraumbilical incision, unless the fibroid lies above the umbilicus when an approach through the ninth left intercostal space in the midclavicular line should be performed.

2 Check under the fibroid by manoeuvring the laparoscope into the deep cul-de-sac. Determine if endometriosis or rectal tenting is present. If it is, open the peritoneum and reflect the rectum down off the posterior vagina to the loose areolar tissue of the rectovaginal space. Incise the vagina superficially between the uterosacral ligaments with a high-power CO_2 laser through the operating laparoscope or with a spatular monopolar electrode. The incision marks the vagina for later entrance and does not penetrate its full thickness, so that the pneumatoperitoneum is maintained.

3 Check ovaries. Remove one at this stage only if the fibroid has

pulled it and its associated ligaments across the midline. In most cases with a very large uterus it is better to preserve the ovaries at the start of the case to avoid problems with the pelvic side-wall. The ovaries should be re-examined when the uterus has been removed, and excised at that time if appropriate.

4   With a large fibroid uterus, the utero-ovarian ligament/round ligament/fallopian tube pedicle is markedly elongated. It is most convenient and quickest to use two Endo GIA 30-staple cartridges to divide this elongated pedicle. Use of this instrument in this circumstance is most helpful in reducing back-bleeding. When bipolar desiccation is used in this situation, troublesome back-bleeding often occurs as the uterus is manipulated, requiring many returns to the bleeding sites for desiccation.

5   The vesicouterine peritoneal fold is divided with scissors, electrosurgical electrode or CO_2 or Nd-YAG laser. This part of the operation is performed after the utero-ovarian/fallopian tube/round ligament complex has been divided because with large fibroids the bladder is far down in the pelvis and the vesicouterine fold is stretched out. With a smaller fibroid uterus, this part may be done prior to firing the Endo GIA.

6   At this stage it is usually possible to incise both the anterior and the posterior vagina laparoscopically and then proceed vaginally. Allen stirrups are changed to candy-cane stirrups and the surgeon then sits between the patient's legs. Vaginal clamps are applied, the uterosacral ligaments, the cardinal ligaments and the uterine vessels are clamped and divided and the sutures are ligated. The uterus is then removed after extensive morcellation.

7   When very large fibroids are located high above the level of the internal os of the cervix, it is often possible to manipulate the laparoscope above or beneath the fibroid into the deep pelvis. The ureters on each side should then be identified, grasped using atraumatic forceps and separated from the uterine vessels, which are separated and ligated in the manner previously described, using a curved-needle technique. The vagina is entered anteriorly and posteriorly and the cardinal ligaments are divided between these two incisions. The free uterus is removed from below after extensive morcellation.

Laparoscopic uterosacral vaginal suspension

It is often possible to improve on the amount of vaginal elevation obtained after hysterectomy by using a laparoscopic technique. When a hysterectomy is being performed vaginally in cases with uterine prolapse, it may be useful to first dissect the ureters laparoscopically and to define the uterosacral ligaments. These can subsequently be secured to the sacrum in a very high position. Curved-suture techniques are used to apply o Vicryl on a CT 1 needle to these firm ligaments immediately adjacent to the upper rectum. The suture material is left long in the peritoneal cavity for subsequent fixation. Following vaginal removal of the uterus, previously applied sutures are grasped with the surgeon's index finger and brought down into the vagina. These sutures are then applied to the vaginal cuff, using a free curved needle, and tied after completion of the vaginal repair. This technique brings the vagina into a higher position than is possible with a conventional technique.

Summary

The principle behind the laparoscopic approach to hysterectomy is becoming clear and it is the desirability of avoiding a large laparotomy scar. To achieve this goal, some of the hysterectomy may be performed laparoscopically and some by the conventional vaginal route. We believe that the proportion of the operation which should be done laparoscopically will vary and should depend on the amount of the operation which can most conveniently, quickly and safely be done from above. Conversely, that which can most effectively and efficiently done from below should be done vaginally. At what stage the transition from one approach to the other takes place will depend on the nature of the pathology, the size of the uterus, the equipment available and the skill and preference of the operator. Each of the laparoscopic stages of the procedure can be performed with a variety of different techniques. There may be little to choose between the results of these various approaches when used by an operator who fully understands the equipment he/she has chosen to use. The most important prerequisite is that the gynaecologist is very familiar with the principles and necessary limitations of abdominal, vaginal and laparoscopic techniques.

Detractors of the concept of laparoscopic hysterectomy argue that vaginal hysterectomy is faster and less expensive and results in a similar short hospital stay and convalescence. However, 75% of all hysterectomies are currently performed abdominally. If laparoscopic hysterectomy is added to the gynaecological armamentarium, almost all hysterectomies may be done without an abdominal incision. We predict that abdominal hysterectomy will become an increasingly rare procedure over the next few years.

The main objective of this book is to help the surgeon achieve the goal of being able to offer his/her patient vaginal hysterectomy, laparoscopic-assisted vaginal hysterectomy or laparoscopic hysterectomy, depending on their clinical need and being able to avoid an abdominal incision without jeopardizing safety. Laparoscopic hysterectomy should not be seen as an exercise in surgical dexterity. If vaginal hysterectomy is easy after securing the utero-ovarian ligaments, it should be done. Laparoscopic inspection at the end of the procedure will still allow the surgeon to control any residual bleeding and evacuate any clot. Unnecessary operations should not be done to satisfy the surgeon's preoccupation with the development of surgical skills and operative techniques. Neither should these procedures be done by those unaware of the necessary reproductive anatomy, the physiology and the clinical manifestation of pelvic disease. Laparoscopic hysterectomy should only be performed when it can offer the patient a less invasive and painful method of achieving relief of her symptoms without increased risk of surgical injury.

Reference

1 Bruhat MA, Mage G, Pouly JL, Manhes H, Canis M, Wattiez A. *Laparoscopic Hysterectomy in Operative Laparoscopy*, pp. 217–221. McGraw-Hill, New York, 1992.

Fig. 6.2 The am
removed with C.

A standard hy:
enucleation of i
new technique
cardinal ligamei
nerves and topc
usually perforn
can be employe

Adopting th
vaginal and abc
(classic abdomi
alter the topogr
original reason
hysterectomy w
cervical stump
1.7% of cases
CASH procedur
the entire transf
the potential fo
removed in tra
Figs 6.1 and 6.2

The advanta

1   Surgical adv.
(a)   A safe
tissues.
(b)   Preservi
(c)   Preservi

surgery using scissors, scalpels and sutures are applied. Throughout the development of pelviscopic surgery, various techniques have been developed to replace the suture techniques for haemostasis. Some of these, such as electrosurgery or laser coagulation, used to excess can produce a 'barbecued lady'. From 1974 I have concentrated on developing pelviscopic techniques which follow the classic modalities of open surgery. I recommend the use of loop ligation and suturing with extra- and intracorporeal knots. These classic techniques can be complemented by the use of endocoagulation using crocodile forceps, which can in some circumstances save time.

This technique is a natural development from my work published in 1984 on pelviscopic salpingo-oophorectomy using the triple-loop ligation technique. In that procedure the infundibulopelvic ligament, the fallopian tube and the suspensory ligament of the ovary were properly and functionally ligated. The creation of the SEMM (serrated-edge macromorcellator) allows large tissue masses to be removed from the abdomen. When the uterus is so debulked, the triple-loop ligation technique can then be used to facilitate a pelviscopic hysterectomy. This technique uses only needles and sutures for haemostasis. High-frequency monopolar or bipolar diathermy and lasers are not used.

Indications for CASH per pelviscopy

A uterus of 12 weeks' size can be morcellated with the SEMM in 10−15 min. Any uterus of this size or less can be removed pelviscopically, even when associated with severe intra-abdominal adhesions or a history of multiple previous laparotomies. A uterus larger than 12 weeks is best removed at open laparotomy but the same CASH principles can be applied.

Preoperative preparation for pelviscopic CASH

The preoperative preparation should be the same as for a patient about to undergo a laparotomy. The patient must be clearly informed and give consent for an immediate laparotomy if this should prove clinically necessary. I recommend that enemas are given on the two days prior to and on the day of surgery to ensure that the bowels are adequately emptied on the day of the operation. This is important as a bowel which is full is a constant disturbance to the operative procedure. It is difficult to keep a full bowel out of the lower pelvis, with the result that if the operating field is not clear the operating time will be prolonged. I also recommend a preoperative intravenous pyelogram to demonstrate the course of the ureters.

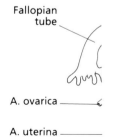

Fallopian
tube

A. ovarica

A. uterina

Ureter

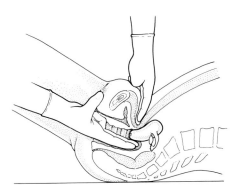

Fig. 6.3 Bimanual palpation of the uterus prior to CASH.

Preparation for cervical excision

It is important that a complete set of instruments is available. The uterus must be palpated manually and its position and the size of the cervix assessed (Fig. 6.3). The diameter of the cervix should also be assessed by preliminary vaginal ultrasound. The correct size of calibrated uterine resection tools (CURT) must then be selected and prepared.

Pelviscopic hysterectomy

The operation begins in accordance with classical principles of laparotomy as regards the preoperative preparation, type of anaesthesia, disinfection of the abdominal wall and vagina, etc. These precautions are essential in case in an emergency it should be necessary to resort to laparotomy. A full laparotomy set of instruments should also be readily available and of course the surgeon should be completely confident of the traditional laparotomy procedures as well as the pelviscopic ones. The possibility of rapid change from pelviscopy to laparotomy gives the surgeon extra security.

Preliminary pelviscopic inspection

The operation begins with the induction of a pneumatoperitoneum, following the 10 security steps of Semm. Then a 5-mm diagnostic telescope is inserted into the umbilical incision. This readily allows a detailed 360° check of the abdomen. The topography of the lower pelvis is checked and the suitability of the case for pelviscopic hysterectomy is confirmed. The diagnostic pelviscope is changed for a 10-mm surgical optic, using the atraumatic dilatation system (Fig. 6.4).

Coring out the cervix and uterine fundus using CURT

The assistant then checks for one last time the diameter of the cervix by manual vaginal examination. Vaginal retractors are then inserted to expose the cervix. The uterine cavity is sounded and the flexion of the uterus determined. The cervical canal is dilated from Hegar 3 to 5 to permit the insertion of the 5-mm perforation probe of the CURT system. This system is composed of three parts (Fig. 6.5):
1 A 5-mm-diameter, 50-cm-long perforation probe.
2 A centralizing cylinder.
3 A serrated-edged macromorcellator.

The cervix seldom measures more than 2.5 cm in diameter and macromorcellators of 10 mm, 15 mm and 20 mm are available. If the transformation is unusually large, the macromorcellator will not be able to remove all the potentially malignant tissues. In such circumstances, a simultaneous cone biopsy can be performed. In more usual

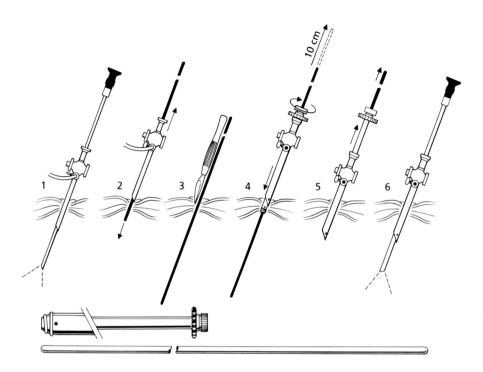

Fig. 6.4 Initial 5-mm diagnostic laparoscopy then atraumatic dilatation system to insert a 10-mm laparoscope.

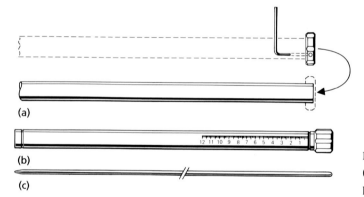

Fig. 6.5 The CURT system. (a) Serrated-edged macromorcellator. (b) A graduated centralizing cylinder. (c) 50-cm long perforating probe.

circumstances, one of the macromorcellators is selected. The 5-mm perforation probe is then inserted into the uterine cavity (Fig. 6.6).

Perforation of the uterine fundus

The surgeon and the assistant must work as a team to control the uterus so that the fundus will be perforated in the proper area. Once the perforation probe is placed in the uterine cavity, its further advancement is controlled under direct pelviscopic vision. The assistant advances the probe into the uterine fundus and the pelviscopic surgeon mobilizes and manipulates the uterus so that a central perforation point is achieved. The surgeon manipulates the uterus using two biopsy or grasping forceps in the closed position. Once the tip of the perforation probe appears in the exact middle of the fundus, the uterus

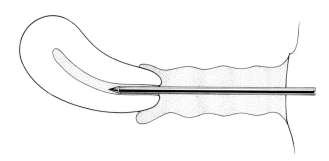

Fig. 6.6 Inserting the perforation probe into the uterus.

is perforated with the tip of the perforation probe. Prior to perforation, the blanching around the tip can easily be seen with the pelviscope and the tip thereby adjusted until in the optimum position. This perforation is performed without blood loss. The perforating rod is then advanced a further 2–3 cm and then secured to the two tenaculums with a special screw forceps (Fig. 6.7).

Separation of the adnexa

When the ovaries are to be removed with the uterus, the next step in the procedure is to ligate the infundibulopelvic ligament. In order to perform this, four 5-mm portals of entry are required. Down one of these is introduced a long, sharp needle, at least 3.5 mm long. This is directed with needle-holders and graspers through the peritoneum below the IP ligament and the suture tied by either extra- or intra-corporeal techniques. The procedure is repeated a short distance medially and then the ligament is divided. Additional haemostatic

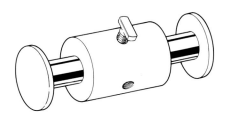

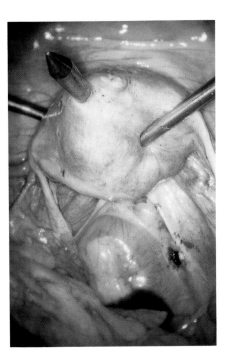

Fig. 6.7 Screw forcep to secure perforating rod to tenaculums.

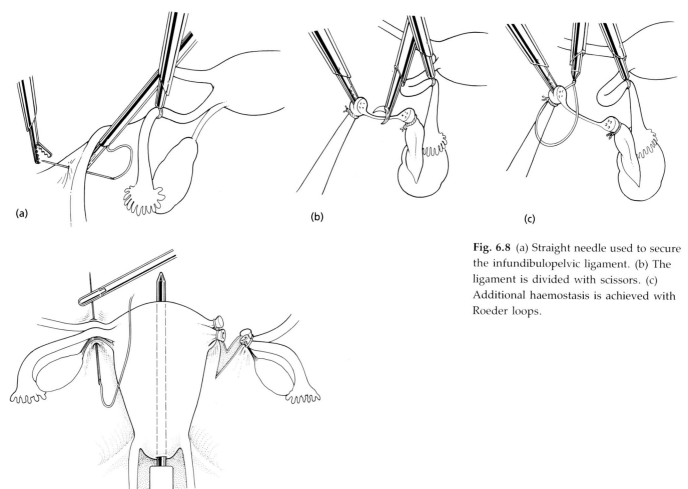

(a)   (b)   (c)

Fig. 6.8 (a) Straight needle used to secure the infundibulopelvic ligament. (b) The ligament is divided with scissors. (c) Additional haemostasis is achieved with Roeder loops.

Fig. 6.9 Position of sutures when ovaries are to be conserved.

security is achieved by also applying a Roeder loop to each side of the pedicle (Fig. 6.8(a)−(c)). Pelviscopic surgery allows careful and close examination of these vessels and the procedure may be completed with very little blood loss.

If the ovaries are to be conserved the suture ligature is placed as shown in Fig. 6.9. Particular care must be taken to locate the large vessels in the broad ligament before inserting this suture so that they may be avoided. After trying two ligatures, the adnexa are separated using scissors. The leaves of the broad ligament can then also be separated.

Establishing intracervical ischaemia

In order to minimize blood loss during the coring-out procedure, we inject 0.05 IU POR in 8 ml of sodium chloride just under the vesicouterine peritoneum into the cervix on each side (Fig. 6.10). This injection also facilitates the separation of the bladder from the upper cervix, which can be achieved using a swab on a special holder (Fig. 6.11).

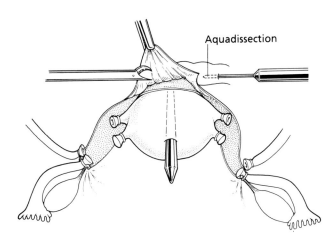

Fig. 6.10 Aquadissection with Pitressin to facilitate separation of the bladder from the upper cervix.

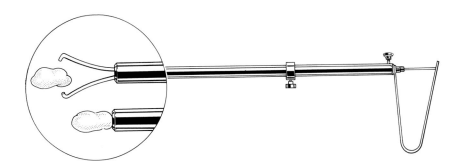

Fig. 6.11 Laparoscopic swab holder.

Suspension of the vesicouterine peritoneum

When the peritoneum and the bladder have been separated sufficiently, the fold of peritoneum is suspended using a 7-cm-long straight CASH needle set. The needle is pushed through the abdominal wall from the outside into the abdominal cavity. It is then passed through the peritoneum a few times and then brought out on the other side once again, going through the whole thickness of the abdominal wall. Both ends of the suture are secured with forceps after being pulled tight. This gives excellent elevation of the vesicouterine peritoneum and thus the bladder, and thereby provides an optimum view for the surgeon (Fig. 6.12).

Triple cervical suture

When the pericervical area has been properly dissected out, a Roeder loop is set over the uterine fundus and is pushed down towards the cervical area (Fig. 6.13). If the uterus is too large for the preformed loop, the endoligature technique with extracorporeal tying can be tried. The ligature is tied at this time to reduce the risk of gas embolism with the CO_2 entering the major uterine vessels when they are subsequently cut.

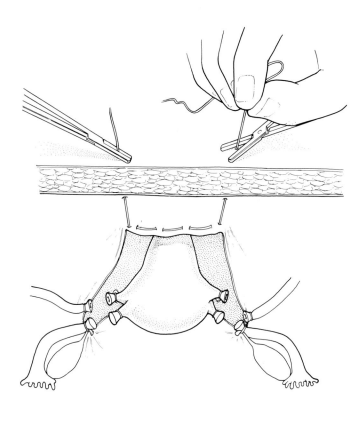

Fig. 6.12 CASH needle set to elevate vesicouterine peritoneum and maximize view of lower pelvis.

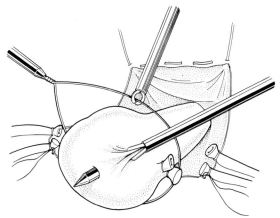

Fig. 6.13 Applying large Roeder loop over uterine fundus.

This technique ensures:
1 No gas loss.
2 All pericervical vessels are ligated.
3 Prevention of gas embolism.

Cervical uterine fundus tissue excision

Once the first Roeder loop has been correctly placed, the tenaculums are released and the CURT is pushed over the perforation probe. This procedure can be done blindly as the cutting element of the CURT is situated 5 mm behind the leading cylinder (see Fig. 6.5). Once the centralizing tool has touched the cervix, the assistant begins turning the cutting cylinder slowly, applying only a little pressure. The quicker the rotating movements, the lower the pressure required to excise the tissue. The length of the cylinder excised can be checked on the graduated scale on the guiding tool. The cutting edge must be very sharp and so the serrated-edged tools are supplied in packets of five and must be replaced as soon as blunted. When the edge of the tool appears at the uterine fundus, the pressure on the instruments should be further reduced and the actual perforation of the fundus should be done very slowly. The procedure is controlled on the video-screen, which is observed by both surgeon and assistant. After the transuterine cylinder has been cored out (Fig. 6.14), the assistant carefully removes, under direct visual control, the tissue cylinder from the uterine cavity. The 10-mm claw forceps now grasps the uterine fundus and the uterus is gently pulled up in the direction of the vagina.

Triple cervical ligature

After the first Roeder loop has been set in the proper position, the macromorcellator is removed from the vagina by the assistant. The endoscopic surgeon then immediately pulls the Roeder loop taut by pushing the knot down with the plastic handle. The surgeon knows the knot is correctly tied when he/she no longer hears the noise of air rushing out of the vagina. If the hissing sound persists, a second tightening of the suture is required. Two further Roeder knots are applied under direct vision of both the anterior aspect of the cervix and the posterior cervix and uterosacral ligaments. Synthetic monofilament sutures are not as safe as catgut for this stage of the operation

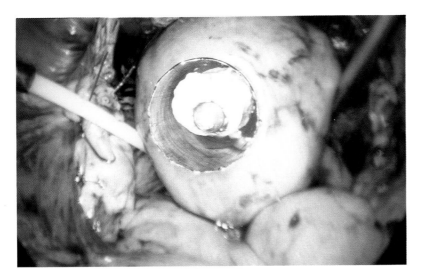

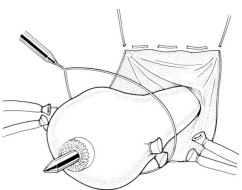

Fig. 6.14 Coring out the uterine cylinder with the Semm macromorcellator.

as the synthetic sutures may slip. Catgut swells with time and this should prevent subsequent slipping. As an additional safety precaution, I recommend applying a fourth Roeder loop when the uterus has been removed.

Haemostasis in the cored-out cervix

The cervical haemostasor is introduced vaginally into the perforation site. This instrument is applied for 2 min at a temperature of 120°C and this ensures adequate haemostasis. When this has been completed the perforation guide and the haemostasor are removed.

Resection of the uterus

When the pericervical tissues have been ligated three times, the uterine corpus is pulled, with the help of the claw forceps, in the direction of the umbilicus. Then, using a hooked scissors or a knife, the cervix is transected (Fig. 6.15).

Temporary fixation of the amputated uterus

When I first started performing the CASH technique, it was my practice to 'park' the uterus for a while in the upper abdomen. However, on one occasion I lost a uterus. This had been parked in the middle of the abdomen. During this exercise the patient strained against the anaesthesia and thereafter the uterus could not be found. The operation was ended and she had repelviscopy 2 days later. We believed the uterus would then be found in the pouch of Douglas. The uterus could not be found and a laparotomy was consequently performed. The uterus was found tucked under the spleen. This very time-consuming procedure caused the additional stress of a second anaesthetic and an unwanted

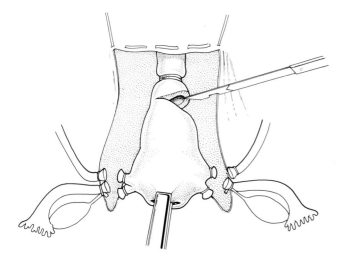

Fig. 6.15 Transecting the uterine fundus from the triple-ligated cervix.

laparotomy. Following this incident, I now consider transabdominal fixation of the amputed uterus as mandatory (Fig. 6.16).

Elevation of the pelvic floor

The round ligaments are next fixed to the cervical stump (Fig. 6.17). A long, sharp needle with slowly resorbable suture material is suggested.

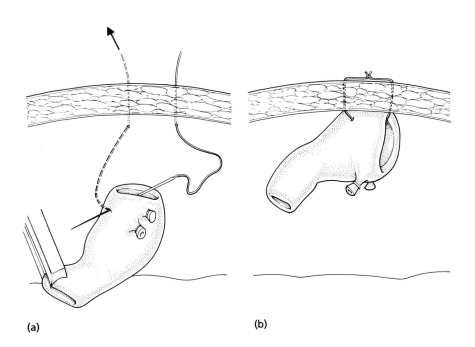

Fig. 6.16 Transabdominal fixation of the amputated uterus.

(a)

(b)

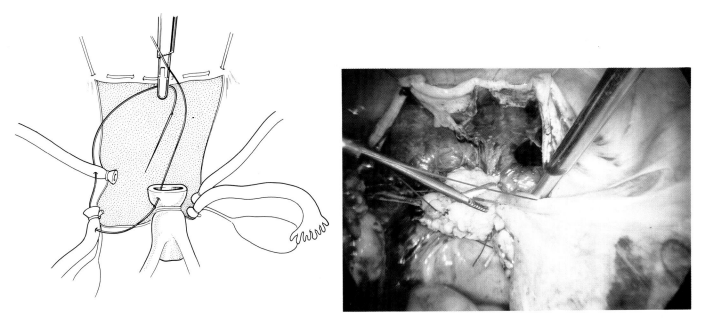

Fig. 6.17 Ligating round ligaments to the cervical stump.

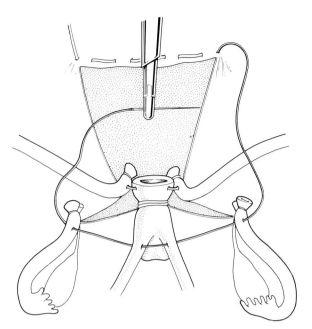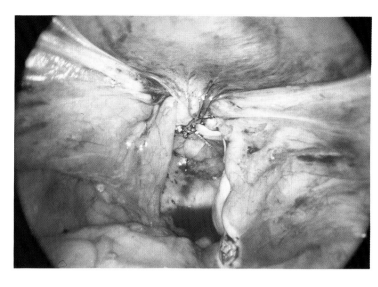

Fig. 6.18 Semm's purse-string suture to reperitonealize the cervical stump.

Reperitonealization of the cervical stump

After the ligaments have been secured to the stump, the operative area is peritonealized. The first step is to cut the suture of the CASH needle set, which is still lying outside the abdomen. This suture is reintroduced into the abdomen once the needle has been cut off extra-abdominally. The short needle is now pulled into the abdomen. This short needle is grasped and inserted through the round ligament and the fallopian tube, and then passed directly through both uterosacral ligaments. This is a type of purse-string suture (Fig. 6.18). Then the short needle is cut off and removed from the abdomen. Both free ends are then tied intracorporeally. The vesicouterine peritoneal fold which the CASH needle set had previously suspended now falls over the cervical stump, like a curtain coming down at the theatre. The lower pelvis is then liberally irrigated with several litres of warmed normal saline (40°C) using the aquapurator.

Morcellating the uterus

This is the final step of the operation. To prepare for morcellation one of the 11-mm suprapubic trocars should be exchanged for a larger 15- or 20-mm one, depending upon the size of the uterus. Morcellation of the uterine corpus, using the big claw forceps of the SEMM, is next performed (Fig. 6.19). The larger trocars should not be used until this stage for there is otherwise a tremendous loss of gas during the operation, making the operative manipulations more difficult.

The pericervical fascia and the pedicles which remain must be

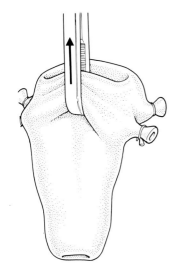

Fig. 6.19 Grasping the uterus prior to morcellation.

completely extraperitonealized. The uterus must be completely morcellated and care taken to ensure that none is left in the abdominal cavity. All blood clots and debris must be removed, remembering to remove fluid from the subphrenic space. This can be done with the new Wisap Bifi suction set. The operative field is then repeatedly bathed and rinsed with normal saline until the fluid remains clear. A 5-mm Robinson's drain is placed down a 5-mm trocar sheath (Fig. 6.20). This is a gravity drain and any fluid left in the abdomen rapidly drains out. An added advantage is that if there is any postoperative bleeding this may be immediately detected. The drain should be removed within 12–24 hours. The trocar skin wounds are closed with staples, which can be removed in 2–3 days.

Postoperative care of the cervical wound

This technique of coagulation of the cervix is derived from my three decades of work in the use of a coagulator for the treatment of cervical

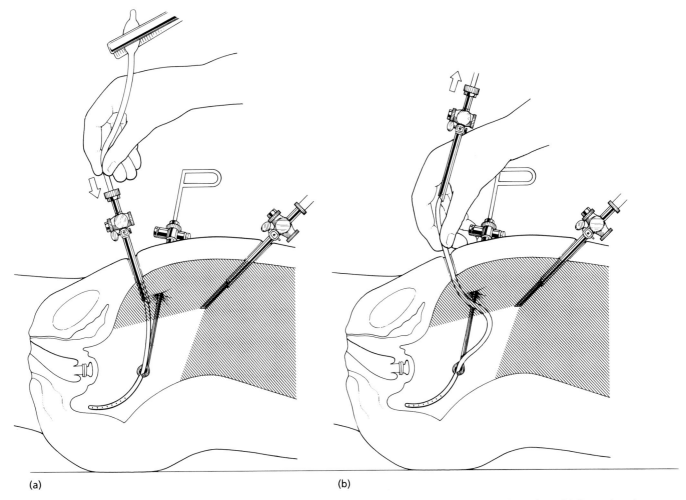

(a)

(b)

Fig. 6.20 (a) Inserting a 5-mm Robinson's drain into the pelvis. (b) Removing the 5-mm trocar sheath to retain drain.

lesions and achieving haemostasis in the bed of the cervix following cone biopsy. The newly developed cervical haemostasor is an ideal instrument to ensure complete postoperative haemostasis. At the end of the hysterectomy, the cervix is exposed with a Semm's speculum. Demonstration of the pericervical excavation may be easily performed with this instrument and it is preferred because it does not mobilize the stump in the lower pelvis. The risk of dislodging the cervical sutures is thereby reduced. Any bleeding can be controlled with a G probe on the cervix coagulator and this process can be repeated in the early postoperative days if there is any secondary bleeding from this area.

Histopathological specimens after CASH

Using CURT a mucosal cylinder is removed which contains the entire ecto- and endocervix, as well as the isthmus and the mucosa of the uterine cavity, including a large part of the myometrium and uterine fundus. Multiple longitudinal sections can be taken from both the ecto- and endocervix. The endometrium is also sectioned in a longitudinal manner and this permits accurate and well-orientated histology of all the uterine tissues.

7: Pelvic Side-wall Dissection, Laparoscopic Lymphadenectomy and Laparoscopic Dissection of the Obliterated Cul-de-sac

Pathology, particularly endometriosis, adhesions and malignancy, can greatly complicate a hysterectomy, whether it is performed by conventional or laparoscopic routes. This chapter describes some advanced techniques which facilitate the performance of a laparoscopic hysterectomy in association with major pelvic pathology.

Anatomy

The anatomy of the pelvic side-wall should be very familiar to the surgeon performing advanced laparoscopic surgery. When operating near the ureter, it is safer to expose it early than to subsequently have to check its position repeatedly. Laparoscopic access to the pelvic side-wall is superior to laparotomy because of the improved and highly magnified view afforded by the laparoscopic image on the video-monitor.

Arterial supply

The common iliac artery bifurcates into the external and internal iliac arteries between 1.5 and 2 cm below the pelvic brim. The left side consistently divides about 0.5 cm lower than the right. The external iliac artery then passes along the pelvic brim to a point beneath the inguinal ligament, midway between the anterior superior iliac spine and the symphysis pubis. The external iliac vein lies partly beneath and medial to it. The pelvic side-wall is supplied by a series of branches from the internal iliac artery and vein. The internal iliac artery usually passes laterally for about 3 cm and then divides into an anterior visceral branch and a posterior parietal branch. Progressing down the pelvic side-wall, the branches of the anterior division most frequently encountered are: (i) the superior vesical artery; (ii) the obliterated hypogastric artery; (iii) the uterine artery; (iv) the vaginal artery; (v) the inferior vesical artery; (vi) the middle rectal artery; (vii) the internal pudendal vessels; and (viii) the superior rectal artery on the left. The uterine artery has six branches. The first is the ureteric artery, the second the descending cervical branch and then, as it coils and ascends the lateral border of the uterus, it gives off four branches to the round ligament, the fundus, the fallopian tube and the ovary.

Ureter

The ureter runs downwards and medially from the kidney on the psoas major muscle in the subserous fascia of the peritoneum. It enters the pelvic cavity, crossing the common iliac vessels at their bifurcation. The right ureter lies to the right of the inferior vena cava and is crossed by the right colic and ileocolic vessels, the small-bowel mesentery and the terminal part of the ileum. The left ureter is crossed by the left colic vessels from the inferior mesenteric vessels and, just above the pelvic brim, passes behind the sigmoid and its mesocolon. In the pelvis, the ureter lies in front of the hypogastric vessels and medial to the obturator, uterine, inferior vesical and middle rectal arteries. The ureter usually forms the posterior boundary of the ovarian fossa and then runs down to the level of the ischial spine, where it turns to pass downwards, forwards and medially towards the bladder in the base of the broad ligament to reach the ureteric canal in the cardinal ligament. Here it accompanies the uterine vessels for about 2 cm before passing beneath them 1.5–2.0 cm from the cervix. It is this area of the ureter that is most frequently damaged during laparoscopic surgery. The ureter then tunnels through the lateral and anterior parts of the cardinal ligament before entering the base of the bladder.

The adventitia or outer fibrous coat of the ureter is divided into an outer network (ureteric sheath) with unconvoluted blood-vessels that anastomose with each other and an inner network containing densely convoluted cork-screw arteries. Small arteries run radially into the adventitia to supply the muscle coat and the mucosa. The pelvic portion of the ureter is richly supplied by branches from the common iliac artery, internal iliac artery, iliolumbar artery, superior gluteal artery, superior and inferior vesical arteries, ovarian artery and middle rectal artery.

Adventitial spaces

Two avascular spaces filled with fat and areolar connective tissue are present on each pelvic side-wall. These are the paravesical and pararectal spaces. Development of the pararectal space is often important in pelvic side-wall dissection. The space is covered by peritoneum lateral to the uterosacral ligament, posterior vagina and rectum. The landmarks for entry into the space are the ureter attached to the medial peritoneum, the internal iliac artery laterally, the sacrum posteriorly and the broad ligament anteriorly.

Procedures requiring pelvic side-wall dissection: ureteric dissection

Pelvic structures can be adherent because of extensive endometriosis, dense adhesions after infection or previous surgery and postradiation fibrosis. Such matting down may obliterate the normal surgical land-marks. If blunt and aquadissection are not effective in mobilizing the pelvic organs, the rectosigmoid colon and the ureters must be mobilized. On the left side, the stuck-down rectosigmoid colon may obscure all the normal structures, including the ovary and ureter. The left side is usually more accessible but may be obscured by the caecum and the small bowel and, on some occasions, even the rectosigmoid colon may also adhere there. In such circumstances, dissection should start well out of the pelvis where the ureters can easily be seen. Initially, this may be above the sacral promontory. On the left side, the ureter will be seen crossing the common iliac vessels beneath branches of the inferior mesenteric vessels. On the right side, the ureter is usually more lateral, crossing the right external iliac artery soon after its origin. The steepest possible Trendelenberg tilt facilitates this procedure. The small-bowel mesentery must also be manipulated up and to the right to maximize the view.

On the left side, dissection begins well out of the pelvis, where the decending colon becomes sigmoid and the sigmoid colon, with its inverted V-shaped mesocolon, traverses the psoas muscle. Using blunt-tipped, saw-toothed scissors, the lateral reflections of this junction in the paracolic gutter and iliac fossa are divided. Using the blunt tip of the scissors and aquadissection, the sigmoid colon is reflected medially, exposing the psoas muscle. Dissection is continued until the external iliac artery is exposed. Starting laterally along this vessel, the ovarian vessels are identified and, as medial progress is made, the ureter is identified, followed by the superior rectal artery. It is safer to expose the ureter, starting at the pelvic brim and continuing down into the pelvis, after the rectosigmoid colon is freed from deep pelvic side-wall structures. Fibrotic tissue between the rectosigmoid and the ureter should be excised. As the dissection continues into the deep pelvis, a rectal probe is passed to delineate further its position and facilitate retraction of the rectosigmoid away from the pelvic side-wall structures.

On the right side, small-bowel and appendiceal adhesions are frequently encountered. Both scissors and CO_2 laser down the operating laparoscope can be used to divide these adhesions. Once the parietal peritoneum has been incised, aquadissection can be used to develop a plane between the peritoneum and small-bowel serosa. Dissection continues with laser and scissors. Atraumatic forceps or suction traction with the aquadissector is used for traction. The external iliac artery is exposed, and the ureter is identified crossing it and traced into the pelvis.

Smooth, blunt-tipped grasping forceps are used to free the ureter from the surrounding areolar tissue. These forceps are opened both parallel to and perpendicular to the ureter to free it. The dissection often continues down into the deep pelvis where the ureter is crossed by the uterine vessels.

Pelvic side-wall dissection markedly increases the safety of a laparoscopic approach to hysterectomy, particularly when ligating the uterine artery. Using the above techniques with laser, scissors and aquadissection, the uterine artery should be skeletonized and then ligated with a staple, suture or bipolar desiccation.

Laparoscopic lymphadenectomy

Dargent and Salvat published a series of 100 panoramic retroperitoneal pelviscopic lymphadenectomies for the staging of endometrial, cervical and ovarian malignancies in 1989 [1]. They performed this procedure by inserting a rigid laparoscope beneath the deep fascia through a midline incision at the pubic hair-line. The deep fascia was first located and opened, using finger dissection through the midline incision. A 10-mm telescope was then inserted through this incision and the retroperitoneal space was distended with carbon dioxide. The bifurcation of the common iliac was located on each side and the obturator nerve was demonstrated. An obturator space lymphadenectomy was then accomplished.

Reich performed a transperitoneal laparoscopic pelvic lymphadenectomy in November 1988 as a staging procedure for ovarian cancer [2]. Querleu, in France, performed the same operation within a week of this as a staging procedure for cervical cancer. He has subsequently reported a series of 39 cases of cervical cancer in which he has removed between three and 22 lymph nodes with no significant morbidity [3]. Laparotomy and radical hysterectomy were performed after the laparoscopy in 32 of the 39 cases. He found 100% sensitivity and specificity in his series, with no unexpected metastatic nodes found at laparotomy. He suggested that stage 1 and 2 cervical cancers could be cured either by vaginal surgery or by brachiotherapy without the need for external radiotherapy. On the other hand, when metastatic nodes are found, radical hysterectomy can be avoided. He believes that the consequent reduction of risks and costs justifies the additional general anaesthesia and the short hospital stay of a diagnostic laparoscopy.

Querleu gained access to the retroperitoneal space via an incision in the peritoneum between the round and infundibulopelvic ligaments bilaterally and then did a laparoscopic-guided dissection of the external iliac vessels, umbilical artery, and obturator nerve. The peritoneum was left open for lymph drainage into the peritoneal cavity, and no lymphocyst occurred. Average operating time was 90 min.

Querleu and Dargent currently manage early stages of cervical cancer by first dissecting out the ureters and marking them with a loose suture [3]. A bilateral lymphadenectomy is then performed and the procedure is completed by doing a Shauta radical vaginal hysterectomy. With this technique, stage 1B cervical cancer is handled without an abdominal incision.

Reich's technique uses an umbilical 10-mm puncture and two 5-mm lower-quadrant punctures [2]. The lower-quadrant trocars are placed just above the pubic hair-line and lateral to the deep epigastric vessels and the rectus muscles, in the manner previously described. The rectosigmoid and caecum are mobilized and displaced upwards to gain access to the retroperitoneal space at the level of the aortic bifurcation, and the nodal tissue is taken from this area. Then the exposed adipose and lymph tissue lateral to the common and external iliac vessels is excised using a CO_2 laser close to the vessels. The ureter is retracted medially throughout the dissection. After mobilization of the medial and under-surface of the external iliac vein, the obturator internus fascia of the pelvic side-wall is identified. At the junction of the external iliac and hypogastric vein, the obturator nerve, covered with adipose tissue, can be isolated and exposed. Lymph-node-bearing adipose tissue is then excised from the obturator fossa. The upper margin of the dissection is the external iliac vein, the lower margin is the hypogastric vein and the pubic bone is the posterior margin. CO_2 laser is used to divide fibrotic attachments and coagulate small vessels. Larger vessels are controlled with bipolar forceps. At the completion of the dissection, underwater inspection is performed. Any further bleeding may be controlled with Vancaille microbipolar forceps, coagulating through the electrolyte solution.

Complications

Reich has found that complications following pelvic side-wall dissection were rare in a consecutive series of over 400 cases and no case required laparotomy. This low complication rate can only be achieved by using a cautious time-consuming approach and taking care to dissect the ureter and pelvic side-wall vessels.

Ureter

Intraoperatively, ureteral integrity can be checked by injecting 5 ml indigo carmine solution intravenously. Elimination of the dye begins soon after the injection, the dye appearing in the urine within 10 min. Full-thickness ureteral injury mandates a urological consultation followed by laparotomy repair or implantation. Gomel and James have, however, described laparoscopic suture repair of this type of injury [4].

An intravenous urogram should be obtained if postoperative flank or pelvic pain is present after laparoscopic pelvic surgery. Thermal injury to a ureter will result in ureteral narrowing or perforation, with the development of hydronephrosis. Treatment during the early phase is often possible by placing a stent in the ureter for 4−8 weeks.

Pelvic side-wall vessel injury

Injury to the external iliac artery or vein and the hypogastric vein mandates laparotomy and immediate repair by a vascular surgeon. The increased intra-abdominal pressure caused by insufflation of CO_2 and the decreased venous pressure caused by the Trendelenberg position, together with the tamponading effect of an accumulating haematoma, may conceal major venous damage. When the pressure gradients return to normal, bleeding may start again and progress, slowly filling the retroperitoneal space and leading to hypovolaemic shock. It is therefore important to examine all exposed vessels at the end of the procedure with the patient supine and blood-pressure back to normal. Pelvic side-wall clots should be removed before confirming complete haemostasis.

Laceration of all other individual blood-vessels on the pelvic side-wall can be controlled laparoscopically with bipolar desiccation, providing the surgeon has isolated the vessel from the ureter and the obturator nerve. The collateral circulation of the pelvic vessels, including those supplying the uterus, is extensive and will prevent ischaemic changes to the organ supplied by the damaged vessel.

Cul-de-sac obliteration

Cul-de-sac obliteration was defined by Sampson as 'extensive adhesions in the cul-de-sac obliterating its lower portion and uniting the cervix or lower portion of the uterus to the rectum' [5]. Cul-de-sac obliteration is usually secondary to endometriosis and it implies the presence of retrocervical, deep fibrotic endometriosis beneath the peritoneum. This endometriosis is located on or in the anterior rectum, posterior vagina, posterior cervix, rectovaginal septum or uterosacral ligaments. Partial cul-de-sac obliteration means that the deep fibrotic endometriosis is severe enough to alter the course of the rectum. With complete cul-de-sac obliteration, the fibrotic endometriosis involves the entire cul-de-sac between the cervicovaginal junction and the rectum. This condition is notoriously difficult to treat; medical therapy is almost always ineffective. Macro- or microsurgical laparotomy is the standard treatment if fertility is to be preserved and, if the bowel is involved, bowel resection is commonly performed. When further fertility is not required, a pelvic clearance with hysterectomy and bilateral salpingo-oophorectomy is usually performed. A problem with this approach is that it is nearly always done as an intrafascial technique, leaving fibrotic endometriosis on the vagina and rectum with the assumption that this residual disease will resolve after castration. Such resolution frequently does not occur and further very difficult surgery may be necessary to treat vaginal cuff or rectal endometriosis.

Reich has described a laparoscopic approach to this most difficult of gynaecological conditions [6]. With his technique, the anterior rectum is first freed down to the loose areolar tissue of the rectovaginal septum, prior to excising and/or vaporizing visible and palpable deep fibrotic endometriosis. This approach can be successful even when anterior rectal muscularis infiltration is present.

Surgical technique

To determine if the cul-de-sac obliteration is partial or complete, a surgical sponge on a ring forceps is inserted into the posterior vaginal fornix. Complete cul-de-sac obliteration is present when the outline of the posterior fornix cannot be seen through the laparoscope. Partial cul-de-sac obliteration is present when there is tenting of the rectum but the protrusion of the forceps in the posterior vaginal fornix between the inverted U of the uterosacral ligaments can still be identified.

When superficial fibrotic, haemorrhagic, peritoneal endometriosis is associated with cul-de-sac obliteration, these deposits should first be excised. This can be done with a superpulse CO_2 laser beam at 35–40 W, an Nd-YAG laser with sculptured sapphire tip at 10–15 W, a needle electrode at 40 W of unipolar cutting current or scissors. An elliptical incision is made in the normal peritoneum surrounding the lesion and the edge lifted upwards. The lesion is then undermined using the pressurized effect of the aquadissector. This pushes the rectum and other vital structures away and facilitates undercutting of the lesion with the laser, diathermy or scissors. After peritoneal excision, the anterior rectal wall is checked and any superficial endometriosis in that area is excised or vaporized.

Deep fibrotic, nodular endometriosis involving the cul-de-sac is then excised from the posterior vagina, rectum, posterior cervix and uterosacral ligaments. Attention is first directed towards complete dissection of the anterior rectum throughout its area of involvement, until the loose areolar tissue of the rectovaginal space is reached. A ring forceps is placed in the posterior vaginal fornix and a modified no. 81 French probe is inserted into the rectum. In addition, a 2 or 3 Simms blunt curette is placed in the endometrial cavity to markedly antevert the uterus and stretch out the cul-de-sac in order to aid in identification. Using the rectal probe as a guide, the rectal serosa is opened at its junction with the cul-de-sac. Careful blunt dissection is then employed, using the aquadissector for both dissection and suction traction. Sharp dissection with laser, diathermy or scissors is also used to complement the blunt dissection, until the rectum is completely free and identifiable below the lesion. It is important not to attempt excision of the deposits of fibrotic endometriosis until the rectal dissection has been completed.

Deep fibrotic lesions are then excised from the uterosacral ligaments, upper posterior vagina (the location of which is continually confirmed by the sponge in the posterior fornix) and posterior cervix. The dissection of the vaginal wall with laser, aquadissection, electrosurgery or scissors usually reveals an endopelvic fascial layer infiltrated with endometriosis and, when this is excised, the normal, soft, pliable upper posterior vaginal wall can be identified underneath. It can be difficult to distinguish fibrotic endometrium from the posterior cervix at the cervicovaginal junction. Frequent palpation using rectovaginal examinations helps to identify occult lesions. Lesions may penetrate deeply into or completely penetrate the vaginal wall. Dissection is still designed to remove all the deposits and, if required, an *en bloc* laparoscopic resection from the cul-de-sac to the posterior vaginal wall. The pneumatoperitoneum can be maintained by inserting and inflating a 30-ml Foley's catheter into the vagina. The posterior vaginal wall can be closed with sutures, either vaginally or laparoscopically.

Endometriotic nodules infiltrating the anterior rectal muscularis can be excised, with the surgeon's, or his/her assistant's, finger in the rectum just beneath the lesion. Sometimes the anterior rectum can be reperitonealized by plicating the uterosacral ligaments and lateral rectal peritoneum across the midline, using 4–0 polydioxanone or polyglactin 910 suture. The suture can be tied extracorporeally and slid down to the operation site. Deep rectal muscularis defects are always closed with sutures.

The operative advantages of cul-de-sac obliteration are easy intra-operative access to the rectum and vagina, a magnification source which is much easier to manipulate than an operating microscope and the ability to perform an underwater examination at the end of the procedure, during which all blood clots can be evacuated and complete haemostasis obtained. The general advantages of laparoscopic surgery are also of course obtained.

Large-bowel injury

If the large bowel is damaged in unprepared patients, laparotomy, peritoneal toilet and repair by a gastrointestinal surgeon should be performed. In a prepared patient, a rent in the rectum can be repaired with 4–0 silk or 4–0 polydioxanone. Stay sutures are placed at the transverse angles of the defect and brought out through the lower-quadrant trocar sleeves, which are then reinserted through the same incision into the peritoneal cavity over the stay suture. After the two-layer closure, Betadine solution is injected through a Foley's catheter, and an underwater examination is performed to check for any leaks, which, if seen, are then reinforced with further studies.

The knowledge that the bowel can be repaired successfully by laparoscopic techniques should increase the confidence of the surgeon operating in the deep pelvis. Single-layer, end-on, continuous suture repair has been reported for colonic anastomosis.

Conclusion

The techniques of pelvic side-wall and cul-de-sac dissection can be learned and applied safely by the expert laparoscopist. The ability to perform these procedures increases the scope and the safety of laparoscopic surgery for major pathology. The recognition that visualization is improved during laparoscopic surgery is of major importance. Pelvic side-wall or cul-de-sac dissection is employed for many indications and using a variety of techniques. Continued advances in levels of skill and technology available will further enhance the surgeon's ability to accomplish this dissection.

References

1 Dargent D, Salvat J. L'envahissement ganglionnaire pelvien. McGraw-Hill, Paris, 1989.
2 Reich H, McGlynn F, Wilkie W. Laparoscopic management of stage 1 ovarian cancer. *J Repro Med* 1990; **35**: 601−605.
3 Querleu D, Leblanc E, Castelain B. Laparoscopic pelvic lymphadenectomy in the staging of early carcinoma of the cervix. *Am J Obstet Gynae* 1991; **164**: 579−581.
4 Gomel V, James C. Intraoperative management of ureteral injury during operative laparoscopy. *Fertil Steril* 1991; **55**: 416.
5 Sampson JA. Perforating hemorrhagic (chocolate) cysts of ovary. *Arch Surg* 1921; **3**: 245.
6 Reich H, McGlynn F, Salvat J. Laparoscopic treatment of cul-de-sac obliteration secondary to retrocervical deep fibrotic endometriosis. *J Repro Med* 1991; **36**: 516−522.

8: Laparoscopic Retropubic Colposuspension (Burch Procedure)

Reported in the literature are more than 100 different kinds of surgical treatments for stress urinary incontinence in women, including anterior colporrhaphy (Kelly plication) [1], retropubic urethropexy (Marshall—Marchetti—Krantz procedure [2], Burch procedure [3]), paravaginal suspension [4], various kinds of needle urethropexy [5—8], and suburethral sling procedure [9]. Furthermore, among these procedures are many modifications, all of which present a somewhat confusing picture for the practising surgeon in choosing a proper surgical procedure for incontinent patients.

However, with better understanding of the pathophysiology of genuine stress urinary incontinence and with more published data available, there seems to be a consensus, especially among gynaecologists, that retropubic colposuspension (Burch procedure) is the surgical treatment of choice for genuine stress urinary incontinence in patients who have an intact urethral sphincteric mechanism but with poor urethral support and a displaced urethrovesical junction [10, 11]. However, the abdominal Burch procedure requires patients to undergo laparotomy; and the poor visibility of the retropubic space complicates the dissection of space of Retzius and mobilization of the bladder and tends to incur more blood loss. Additional disadvantages include prolonged operating time and increased surgical morbidity.

On the other hand, the various kinds of needle urethropexy can be performed easily with a short operating time and hospital stay. However, most reports in the literature indicate that the long-term results do not appear to be as effective as retropubic colposuspension [12—15]. In our own experience with laparoscopic retropubic colposuspension, there has been minimal blood loss, low morbidity and shortened hospital stay and postoperative recovery. This procedure can conveniently be performed with a laparoscopic hysterectomy when the patient presents with both uterine problems and urinary stress incontinence.

Preoperative evaluation

The diagnosis of genuine stress incontinence must first be confirmed and detrusor instability excluded. The preoperative evaluation includes a complete history and physical examination, with particular emphasis on neurological history and details of current medication. The consultant's incontinence questionnaires and patient's urinary voiding diary (urolog) can add valuable information. Pelvic examination and lower neurological examination, with emphasis on the sensory and motor dermatome pattern of S_2, S_3 and S_4, are also necessary. The examination is supplemented by office investigations, including urinalysis and urine culture, a stress test and a Q-tip test, as well as a simple office cystometry [16] and measurement of residual urine. If there is any abnormality in these tests or if the patient has had previous failed incontinence surgery, she should undergo more sophisticated multichannel electronic urodynamic studies before any treatment is selected.

Operative techniques

Under general anaesthesia with endotracheal intubation, the patient is placed in a low lithotomy position with legs supported in Allen's stirrups (Allen Medical, Mayfield, OH). A no. 20 French sized Foley catheter with a 30-ml balloon tip is then inserted into the bladder, and 50 ml concentrated indigo carmine dye is instilled into the bladder. The Foley catheter is then clamped. Inadvertent penetration of the bladder during the procedure will immediately be revealed by the escape of blue dye. A 10-mm laparoscope is inserted through a vertical intra-umbilical incision, and four 5-mm puncture sites are made in the abdomen (Fig. 8.1). The lower pair of puncture sites is made lateral to the deep inferior epigastric vessels, and the upper pair is placed lateral to the rectus muscle at about the umbilical level. Careful inspection is made of the internal viscus, after which the patient is then placed in a 20° Trendelenberg position, and the pelvic organs are then meticulously examined. All visible pathologies, such as adhesions and endometriosis, are excised, as described in the previous chapter, and the uterus, with or without the ovaries, is laparoscopically removed, as described in Chapter 5. After the vaginal cuff has been closed, the pelvic area is irrigated with copious amounts of Ringer's lactate solution. Underwater examination of the surgical sites is performed to ensure satisfactory haemostasis. The cul-de-sac is then obliterated, using 2−0 permanent sutures, with either the Halban or Moschcowitz procedure, through the laparoscope. The Halban procedure [17] consists of placing several

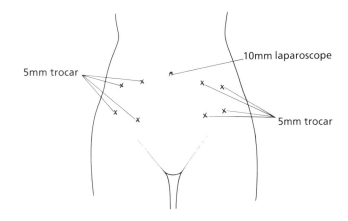

Fig. 8.1 Liu's recommended trocar placements.

sagittal sutures within the cul-de-sac, and the Moschcowitz procedure [18] involves placing one or more purse-string sutures to obliterate the cul-de-sac. It is important to obliterate the channels on either side of the sigmoid colon in both procedures. Either procedure, if properly executed, can prevent future enterocele formation.

1 The laparoscopic retropubic colposuspension proper begins with an incision made about 1 inch above the symphysis pubica in the anterior wall peritoneum. This should be made laparoscopically between the two obliterated bladder folds with laparoscopic scissors.

2 The anterior peritoneum is dissected away from the anterior abdominal wall and the retropubic space is entered.

3 The bladder is mobilized and paravaginal tissue is identified. The fatty tissue around the paravaginal areas is removed and haemostasis achieved with bipolar forceps. No dissection is performed within 2–2.5 cm of the urethra.

4 Two sutures of non-absorbable material are used to raise and pull the anterior vaginal wall forward to the Cooper's ligament. The sutures are inserted at the level of the mid-urethra and the urethrovesical junction. The sutures are inserted at least 2 cm from the urethra. A double bite of the whole thickness of the vagina, avoiding the vaginal cavity, is taken and is then passed through the Cooper's ligament on the ipsilateral side at a level immediately above the location in the anterior vaginal wall. During the insertion of this suture the assistant places his/her middle and index fingers at the level of the urethrovesical junction. Tenting of the anterior vaginal wall in this manner facilitates the correct placement of the sutures. Once the suture has been correctly placed, it can be tied using the extracorporeal technique with the Clarke–Reich knot-pusher [19] previously described. Tying is facilitated if the assistant pushes the fingers in the vagina up towards the Cooper's ligament. The procedure is then repeated on the contralateral side.

During the tying of the knots, particular care must be taken to avoid compressing or kinking the urethra. It is not necessary to have the vaginal wall in direct contact with the Cooper's ligament and adequate support will be obtained if the sutures are snugly tied without undue tension. Excessive tension will produce necrosis at the suture sites and may result in suture release and surgical failure.

5 The retropubic space is then irrigated with copious amounts of Ringer's lactate solution. Any bleeders are coagulated with bipolar forceps.

6 A suprapubic catheter is inserted into the bladder under direct visualization. The peritoneal defect is closed with 2–0 absorbable suture.

7 Cystoscopic examination is then performed to ensure that no suture material has penetrated the bladder wall. To confirm the integrity of the ureters, 5 ml of indigo carmine dye and 20 mg of furosemide (Lasix) may then be injected intravenously.

Postoperative care

The postoperative care is similar to that given after a standard laparoscopic hysterectomy. The majority of patients can be discharged from the hospital within 24 hours of surgery with some mild analgesic medication. These patients, however, will go home with an indwelling suprapubic catheter, which can be removed at the 1-week postoperative check. They are taught self-catheterization and given six disposable plastic catheters to take home with them. With this regime, we have little problem with postoperative voiding difficulties. This postoperative management programme is effective in the US, but in Britain and most of Europe it is probable that the patient and doctor would prefer the patient to remain in the hospital until she is voiding spontaneously without problems.

Complications

The most common complications of open retropubic urethropexy and colposuspension procedures are retropubic haematoma, abscess, wound infection, urinary tract injury, development of detrusor instability, enterocele and sexual dysfunction. With laparoscopic techniques, the space of Retzius can be clearly seen in a much magnified form on the video-monitors. With such excellent vision, the dissection of the space of Retzius and mobilization of the bladder become easier. Haemostasis is also easier and the procedure can be practically bloodless. This in turn helps the surgeon to more accurately place the sutures in the paravaginal fascia and Cooper's ligament.

A particular hazard during an open Burch procedure is damage to the aberrant obturator veins. These veins appear to be consistently present and can easily be avoided when identified with the laparoscope. No significant bleeding occurred in a series of more than 60 cases of laparoscopic retropubic colposuspensions and in no case was it necessary to use a drain.

Summary

The laparoscopic techniques described here closely follow the principles for a Burch procedure proposed by Dr E.A. Tanagho [20]. These include avoiding dissection within 2 cm of the urethra, removing all the fatty tissue in the paravaginal area, avoiding kinking or strangulating the urethra and tying the sutures without undue tension.

To date about 5% of my patients have developed postoperative detrusor instability. All of these had a negative Q-tip test and their symptoms improved with oxybutynin (Ditropan) and bladder retraining. It is not clear if these cases were caused by the surgery or were not detected in the preoperative assessment. Although the majority of failures of anti-incontinence surgery occur within the first 2 years after the procedure, the failure rate increases with time. I have been performing laparoscopic retropubic colposuspensions for the past 2 years and, although my series is still small, I remain encouraged by the results. Patients who have a laparoscopic procedure have less discomfort, much less blood loss, a shorter hospital stay and a quicker recovery time than patients treated with a similar procedure through an abdominal incision. I believe laparoscopic retropubic colposuspension can be a satisfactory alternative to abdominal retropubic colposuspension in well-selected cases and it can be conveniently performed at the same time as a laparoscopic hysterectomy.

References

1 Kelly HA, Dumm WM. Urinary incontinence in women without manifest injury to the bladder: a report of cases. *Surg Gynecol Obstet* 1914; **18**: 444.

2 Marshall VF, Marchetti AA, Krantz KE. The correction of stress incontinence by simple vesicourethral suspension. *Surg Gynecol Obstet* 1949; **88**: 590.

3 Burch JC. Urethrovaginal fixation to Cooper's ligament for correction of stress incontinence, cystocele and prolapse. *Am J Obstet Gynecol* 1961; **81**: 281.

4 Richardson AC, Edmonds PB, Williams NL. Treatment of stress urinary incontinence due to paravaginal fascia defect. *Obstet Gynecol* 1981; **57**: 357–362.

5 Pereyra AJ, Lebherz TB. Combined urethrovesical suspension and vaginourethroplasty for correction of urinary stress incontinence. *Obstet Gynecol* 1967; **30**: 537.

6 Raz S. Modified bladder neck suspension for female stress incontinence. *Urology* 1981; **17**: 82.

7 McGuire EJ, Lyton B. Pubovaginal sling procedure for stress incontinence. *Surg Gynecol Obstet* 1973; **136**: 547.

8 Gittes RF, Loughlin KR. No-incision pubovaginal suspension for stress incontinence. *J Urol* 1987; **138**: 568.

9 Hohnfellner R, Petrie E. Sling procedures in surgery. In: Stanton SL, Tanagho E (eds) *Surgery of Female Incontinence*, 2nd edn, pp. 105–113. Springer-Verlag, Berlin, 1986.

10 Bergman A, Ballard C, Koonings P. Primary stress urinary incontinence and pelvic relaxation: prospective randomized comparison of three different operations. *Am J Obstet Gynecol* 1989; **161**: 97–101.

11 Bergman A, Ballard C, Koonings P. Comparison of three different surgical procedures for genuine stress incontinence: prospective randomized study. *Am J Obstet Gynecol* 1989; **160**: 1102–1106.

12 Karram MM, Bhatia NN. Transvaginal needle bladder neck suspension procedures for stress urinary incontinence: a comprehensive review. *Obstet Gynecol* 1989; **73**: 906–914.

13 Bhatia NN, Bergman A. A modified Burch versus Pereyra retropubic urethropexy for stress urinary incontinence. *Obstet Gynecol* 1980; **66**: 255.

14 Mundy AR. A trail comparing the Stamey bladder neck suspension procedure with colposuspension for the treatment of stress incontinence. *Br J Urol* 1983; **55**: 687–690.

15 Green DF, McGuire EJ, Lytton B. A comparison of endoscopic suspension of the vesical neck versus anterior urethropexy for the treatment of stress urinary incontinence. *J Urol* 1986; **136**: 1205–1207.

16 Walters M, Shields L. The diagnosis value of history, physical examination and the Q-tip cotton swab test in women with urinary incontinence. *Am J Obstet Gynecol* 1988; **159**: 145–149.

17 Halban J. *Gynäkologische Operationslehre*. Urban & Schwarzenberg, Berlin and Vienna, 1932.
18 Moschcowitz AV. The pathogenesis, anatomy, and cure of prolapse of the rectum. *Saxgynecol Obstet* 1912; **15**: 7−21.
19 Reich H, Clarke C. A simple method for ligating with straight and curved needles in operative laparoscopy. *Obstet Gynecol* 1992; **79**: 143−147.
20 Tanagho EA. Colpocystourethropexy: the way we do it. *J Urol* 1976; **116**: 751−753.

9: Laparoscopic Supracervical Hysterectomy

Total abdominal hysterectomy, as described by Dr Richardson in 1929, was introduced in an attempt to control the incidence of cervical cancer. The greater technical difficulties and operative dangers associated with this approach were felt to be outweighed by the need to reduce the incidence of this potentially fatal neoplasm. The operatively easier supracervical approach accordingly fell into disrepute. Cutler, however, reported in 1949 that the incidence of cervical stump carcinoma following supracervical hysterectomy in 6600 cases was only 0.4%. Kikku from Finland reported a postsupracervical hysterectomy stump carcinoma rate of 0.11%. This rate is similar to the rate of vaginal cancer occurring after total hysterectomy. The Finnish group also reported a number of other advantages of subtotal hysterectomy, including decreased urinary tract symptomatology, decreased dyspareunia, decreased bowel symptomatology and, most importantly, decreased injury to ureter and bladder. As the morbidity and operative time of a laparoscopic supracervical hysterectomy is likely to be lower than after a total laparoscopic procedure, it was felt that the supracervical approach should be re-evaluated.

Preoperative preparation

Patient preparation

The patient is positioned for exploratory laparotomy in the modified dorsal lithotomy position with lower limbs in Allen stirrups. The patient is advised of the possible need to convert the procedure to a total or an open type of hysterectomy. She is also fully counselled about the potential risks of retaining the cervix. General anaesthesia with endotracheal intubation is induced and the patient initially placed in a flat position.

The primary umbilical trocar is inserted by the open Hasson technique previously described. A 10-mm Hasson cannula or disposable open trocar (Ethicon) is used. A 5-mm secondary trocar is placed suprapubically lateral to each rectus muscle and a 10–12-mm trocar is placed in the midline three to four finger-breadths above the symphysis. Exploratory laparoscopy is performed, pathology is identified and if necessary preliminary adhesiolysis is performed. The ureter is then carefully identified and, when clearly defined, the infundibulopelvic ligaments are desiccated with bipolar electrosurgery. The desiccated area is then divided, either with the Nd-YAG laser scalpel at 10–15 W of power or with sharp laparoscopic scissors. The pedicles may also be ligated with an endoloop of o-PDS, and any residual back-bleeding is controlled with bipolar desiccation. If the pedicles cannot be desiccated, ligatures can be passed and the sutures tied with the extracorporeal knotting technique. The round ligaments are then desiccated and divided in a similar manner. The uterovesical fold is then opened, using the Nd-YAG laser scalpel or scissors, and with blunt and sharp dissection the bladder flap is carefully formed. This is a most important step in the procedure for, when correctly performed, it opens out the uterine fossa to permit subsequent dissection of the uterine vasculature. Aquadissection in this area is frequently difficult or impossible because of dense adhesions, often following caesarean sections; moreover, excessive use of aquadissection in this area may make identification of the uterine arteries and ureter difficult and this dissection technique should be used only sparingly. The posterior leaf of the broad ligament is dissected, allowing the ureter to fall away laterally. After the uterine arteries have been carefully dissected and the ureter again identified, well clear of these structures, the uterine artery is then secured with bipolar desiccation and divided. Ligatures or ligaclips can be used if a satisfactory pedicle can be developed. After dividing the major vessels, the uterus will become increasingly cyanotic and this colour change indicates that it is safe to proceed to the next step of the operation. The Nd-YAG laser scalpel is then usually used to cut down on to the Cohn cannula, which was placed in the cervix preoperatively. A needle cautery or the Harmonic scalpel can also be used to amputate the uterus from the lower cervix. The level of this incision should be placed well below the endocervical os and points down to the ectocervical os to form an inverted cone. The Cohn cannula is then removed and the remainder of the dissection is performed to complete a reverse cone.

After separation of the uterus, the cuff is inspected and any areas of bleeding are coagulated using an appropriate-shaped tip and the Nd-YAG contact system or desiccated with bipolar diathermy. The anterior and posterior folds of the perineum are plicated over the cervical stump using an interrupted mattress suture of 2−o Vicryl or by inserting a series of staples using an endoscopic stapler. Prior to peritoneal closure the endocervical canal can be ablated using the Nd-YAG laser or the monopolar diathermy ball to decrease postoperative leucorrhoea and reduce the risk of dysplasia. The cavity is then copiously irrigated and inspected for signs of bleeding with the intra-abdominal pressure reduced to <8 mmHg. Any bleeding points are coagulated with bipolar diathermy or the Nd-YAG laser haemostatic tip.

The uterus is then morcellated using sharp dissection with the Nd-YAG laser scalpel and large scissors. When cut into a suitable size, the portions of uterus are removed through the open laparoscopy port in the umbilicus. The incision at this site can easily be extended if necessary to accommodate larger specimens. During the specimen extraction, the laparoscope is moved to the lower midline port to permit direct visualization of this stage of the operation. A posterior culdoplasty can be performed at this time by plicating the uterosacral stumps with 2–0 or 0 Vicryl SH suture tied extracorporeally.

After the end of the procedure, the Foley's catheter which was inserted prior to the operation is removed when the patient is ambulatory. Discharge home is accomplished in 18–36 hours. Patients are allowed to return to normal domestic activities in 2–3 days and are able to return to work in 7–10 days. There is no evidence of significant discharge postoperatively and intercourse may be resumed in 2 weeks.

A variation of this technique has been suggested by Professor Donnez of Brussels. Prior to laparoscopy he removes a cylinder of the endocervical canal containing the whole of the transformation zone with the CO_2 laser. He then proceeds laparoscopically in a manner similar to that described above and secures the vascular pedicles with bipolar diathermy. He transects the upper portion of the cervix with needle diathermy and, after securing haemostasis with mono- and bipolar diathermy, he opens the pouch of Douglas from the vagina and delivers the uterus through this posterior colpotomy. If the uterus is enlarged, it is morcellated to complete the delivery of the specimen. The vaginal incision is then closed with two or three interrupted sutures, which can also be inserted through the uterosacral ligaments to increase the amount of support to the vault.

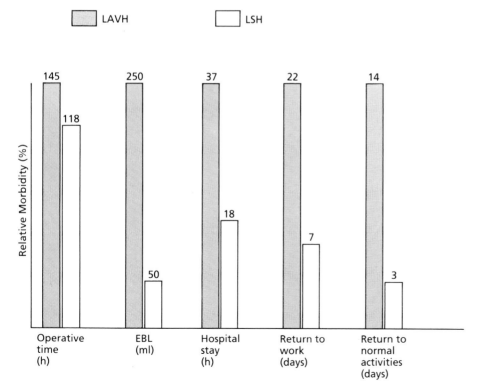

Fig. 9.1 Comparative morbidity of laparoscopic assisted vaginal hysterectomy with laparoscopic supracervical hysterectomy.

The patient's acceptance of laparoscopic supracervical hysterectomy (LSH) is excellent and is associated with a shorter operating time, less peroperative blood loss, a shorter hospital stay, a quicker return to normal household activities and a quicker return to work (Fig. 9.1). Laparoscopic supracervical hysterectomy can be technically easier than laparoscopic hysterectomy. It avoids the risk of adding a difficult vaginal procedure to a difficult laparoscopic procedure. With removal of the transformation zone and regular cytological screening, the risk of stump carcinoma should be very low. It has also been suggested that retaining the cervix retains the possibility of cervical orgasm at subsequent intercourse. For these reasons, this laparoscopic version of an open procedure which fell into disrepute should be reassessed by patients and surgeons contemplating laparoscopic hysterectomy.

Further reading

Ananth J. Hysterectomy and depression. *Obstet Gynecol* 1978; **52** (6): 724−730.

Crossen HS, Crossen RJ. *Operative Gynecology*. C.V. Mosby, St Louis, 1938.

Cutler EC, Zollinger RM. *Atlas of Surgical Operations*. Macmillan Co., New York, 1949.

Dennerstein L, Wood C, Burrows GD. Sexual response following hysterectomy and oophorectomy. *Obstet Gynecol* 1977; **49**: 92.

Dicker RC, Greenspan JR, Strauss LT, *et al*. Complications of abdominal and vaginal hysterectomy among women of reproductive age in the United States. *Am J Obstet Gynecol* 1982; **144**: 841.

Dicker RC, Scally MJ, Greenspan JR, *et al*. Hysterectomy among women of reproductive age: trends in the United States, 1970−1978. *JAMA* 1982; **248**: 323.

Gath D, Cooper P, Bond A, Edmonds G. Hysterectomy and psychiatric disorder. II. Demographic psychiatric and physical factors in relation to psychiatric outcome. *Br J Psychiatry* 1982; **140**: 343−350.

Hoffman MS, Roberts WS, LaPolla JP, Sterghos S, Jr, Cavanagh D. Neoplasia in vaginal cuff epithelial inclusion cysts after hysterectomy. *J Reprod Med* 1989; **34** (6): 412−414.

Johnson CG, Moll CF, Post L. An analysis of 6891 hysterectomies for benign pelvic disease. *Am J Obstet Gynecol* 1956; **71**: 515.

Kikku P. Supravaginal uterine amputation vs. hysterectomy: effects on coital frequency and dyspareunia. *Acta Obstet Gynecol Scand* 1983; **62**: 141.

Kikku P. Supravaginal uterine amputation vs. hysterectomy with reference to subjective bladder symptoms and incontinence. *Acta Obstet Gynecol Scand* 1985; **64**: 375.

Kikku P, Hirvonen T, Gronroos M. Supravaginal uterine amputation vs. abdominal hysterectomy: the effects on urinary symptoms with special reference to pollakiuria, nocturia and dysuria. *Maturitas* 1981; **3**: 197.

Kikku P, Grourros M, Hirvonen T, *et al*. Supravaginal uterine amputation vs. hysterectomy: effects on libido and orgasm. *Acta Obstet Gynecol Scand* 1983; **62**: 147.

Kikku P, Gronroos M, Rauramo L. Supravaginal uterine amputation with preoperative electrocoagulation of endocervical mucosa. *Acta Obstet Gynecol* 1985; **64**: 175.

Kovac SR, Christie SJ, Bindbeutel, GA. Abdominal vs. vaginal hysterectomy: a statistical model for determining physician decision making and patient outcome. *Med Decis Making* 1991; **11** (1): 19−28.

Kraaimaat FW, Veeninga AT. Life stress and hysterectomy−oophorectomy. *Maturitas* 1984; **6** (4): 319−325.

Langer R, Neuman M, Rouel R, *et al*. The effect of total abdominal hysterectomy on bladder function in asymptomatic women. *Obstet Gynecol* 1989; **74**: 205.

Miller NF. Hysterectomy: therapeutic necessity or surgical racket? *Am J Obstet Gynecol* 1946; **51**: 804.

Novak ER, Jones GS, Jones HW. *Novak's Textbook of Gynecology*. Williams and Wilkins, Baltimore, 1965.

Pratt JH. Common complications of vaginal hysterectomy: thoughts regarding their prevention and management. *Clin Obstet Gynecol* 1976; **19**: 645.

Pratt JH. Vaginal hysterectomy by morcellation. *Mayo Clin Proc* 1978; **43**: 374.

Pratt JH, Daikoku ND. Obesity and vaginal hysterectomy. *J Reprod Med* 1990; **35** (10): 945−949.

Pratt JH, Galloway JR. Vaginal hysterectomy in patients less than 36 and more than 60 years of age. *Am J Obstet Gynecol* 1965; **93**: 812.

Pratt JH, Jefferies JA. The retained cervical stump: a 25-year experience. *Obstet Gynecol* 1976; **48**: 711.

Quinlan D, Stutzman R. Flank pain and hematuria following hysterectomy. *Br J Urol* 1987; **60** (4): 371−372.

Reich H, DeCaprio J, McGlynn F. Laparoscopic hysterectomy. *J Gynecol Surg* 1989; **5** (2): 213.

Richardson EH. A simplified technique for abdominal panhysterectomy. *Surg Gynecol Obstet* 1929; **48**: 248.

Sand PK, Bowen LW, Ostergard DR, *et al.* Hysterectomy and prior incontinence surgery as risk factors for failed retropubic cystourethropexy. *J Reprod Med* 1988; **33**: 171.

Siddall RS, Mack HC. Subtotal versus total hysterectomy. *Surg Gynecol Obstet* 1935; **60**: 102.

Sloan D. The emotional and sexual aspects of hysterectomy. *Am J Obstet Gynecol* 1978; **131**: 598.

Snooks SJ, Badenoch DF, Tiptaft RC, *et al.* Perineal nerve damage in genuine stress urinary incontinence. *Br J Urol* 1985; **57**: 422.

TeLinde RW. *Operative Gynecology*. Lippincott, Philadelphia, 1992.

Tervila L. Carcinoma of the cervical stump. *Acta Obstet Gynecol Scand* 1963; **42**: 200.

Utian WH. Effect of hysterectomy, oophorectomy and estrogen therapy in libido. *Int J Gynecol Obstet* 1975; **13**: 97.

Vervest HA, Kiewiet de Jonge M, Vervest TM, Barents JW, Haspels AA. Micturition symptoms and urinary incontinence after non-radical hysterectomy. *Acta Obstet Gynecol Scand* 1988; **67** (2): 141−146.

10: Laparoscopic Dissection of the Pelvic Retroperitoneum and Ureters: Relevant Surgical Anatomy

The peritoneum is draped like a cape over the pelvic organs. Between the peritoneum above, the levator muscles below and the pelvic side-walls laterally, loosely packed fibrous tissue and fat surround the pelvic organs and allow them to distend as necessary. Pelvic ligaments divide this subperitoneal space into six compartments or 'spaces' (Fig. 10.1). The pelvic ureters and major blood-vessels of the pelvis lie in the pararectal and paravesical spaces, and proper development of these spaces is essential to dissection of the pelvic retroperitoneum. In this chapter, the anatomy of the pararectal and paravesical spaces and techniques for opening them at laparotomy and laparoscopically will be described, and their use in identifying vital structures, particularly the ureters, will be discussed.

The pararectal space

If an imaginary line is drawn vertically along the medial leaf of the broad ligament all the way down to the levator floor, the line will successively cross the infundibulopelvic ligament, the ureter, the uterosacral ligament and, finally, the rectal pillars. The pararectal spaces that are used for pelvic surgery are bounded laterally by the internal iliac arteries and medially by the ureters. Before these tissue planes are opened, the ureters lie just above the internal iliac arteries on the pelvic side-wall; after the pararectal spaces are developed, the ureters mark their medial borders. Therefore, development of the pararectal

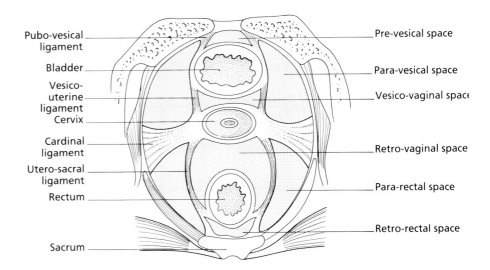

Fig. 10.1 The retroperitoneal pelvic spaces.

Pubo-vesical ligament

Bladder

Vesico-uterine ligament

Cervix

Cardinal ligament

Utero-sacral ligament

Rectum

Sacrum

Pre-vesical space

Para-vesical space

Vesico-vaginal space

Retro-vaginal space

Para-rectal space

Retro-rectal space

spaces always provides a reliable method of identifying the pelvic course of the ureters.

The best way to understand the pararectal space, however, is not from a formal anatomical description but by actually opening the space during an abdominal hysterectomy. This is done in the following manner. First, the broad ligament is opened by dividing the round ligament and incising the peritoneum in a cephalad direction, parallel to the infundibulopelvic ligament up to the pelvic brim. The broad ligament can then be opened bluntly by traction on its medial leaf. This manoeuvre will separate the loose areolar tissue between the leaves of the broad ligament, but an impasse will eventually be reached at about the level of the ureter and internal iliac artery, where the areolar tissue is more condensed and will not separate any further (Fig. 10.2). This point lies at the base of the broad ligament and marks the roof of the pararectal space. Once the pararectal space is opened, it will, of course, be contiguous with the broad ligament.

The external iliac artery is now palpated and traced proximally to the bifurcation of the common iliac artery, so that the internal iliac artery can be clearly felt. The index finger is then placed just medial to the internal artery and pulled inferomedially in the direction of the patient's contralateral femoral head. As this manoeuvre is carried out, a bloodless plane will open up, and the surgeon will find the ureter in his or her dissecting finger. The space will extend from the broad ligament superiorly all the way to the pelvic floor, and will have the following landmarks: the internal artery laterally, the cardinal ligament anteriorly (i.e. caudad), and the ureter, uterosacral ligaments and rectal pillars medially (Fig. 10.3).

Quite frequently, especially in thin, young patients, the dense connective tissue forming the roof of the pararectal space cannot be

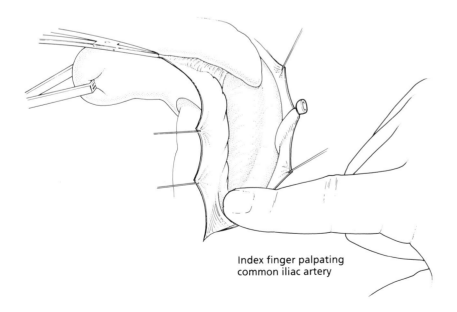

Index finger palpating
common iliac artery

Fig. 10.2 The broad ligament has been opened. The common iliac artery is palpated to locate the internal iliac artery.

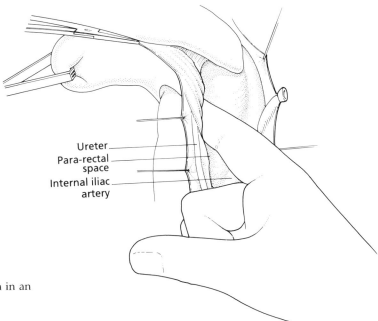

Ureter
Para-rectal space
Internal iliac artery

Fig. 10.3 The pararectal space has been opened by traction in an inferomedial direction, towards the patient's contralateral femoral head. The ureter is against the dissecting finger.

disrupted bluntly, and a small opening must first be made in it with the point of a tonsil clamp or dissecting scissors as the tissue is held taut by medial traction with the dissecting finger. Once a small opening is made, the index finger is insinuated into the pararectal space, which will readily open up if its medial wall is retracted in an inferomedial direction, as previously described. The dense areolar tissue at the base of the broad ligament may be likened to cellophane covering a box. It is difficult to disrupt the cellophane by simply pushing down on it, but, once a small nick is made, the cellophane will spread effortlessly if traction is applied.

It is as well to be aware that another avascular tissue plane can be developed *medial* to each ureter and uterosacral ligament, but lateral to the peritoneum, which forms the medial portion of the broad ligament and its inferior extension into the cul-de-sac. It is this plane which the general surgeon calls the pararectal space and which he/she uses for carrying out either anterior or abdominoperineal resection of the rectum for carcinoma. In other words, our colleagues in general surgery never work laterally to the ureter when performing their pelvic operations but leave it attached in its natural position on the lateral pelvic sidewall.

The paravesical space

The paravesical space is bordered distally or caudad by the pubic bone, proximally or cephalad by the cardinal ligament, medially by the obliterated umbilical artery (also called the lateral umbilical ligament), laterally by the external iliac vessels and inferiorly by the obturator fossa. This space can be easily developed by running the index finger along the medial border or the external iliac artery in a caudad direction until the pubic ramus is reached. Upon reaching the pubic ramus, the direction of the dissection changes abruptly through 90° and is again directed medially towards the patient's contralateral femoral head. A large bloodless plane will again open up, which is the paravesical space, and a cord-like structure will be found in the dissecting finger, which is the lateral umbilical ligament* or obliterated hypogastric artery (Fig. 10.4). The paravesical space usually only needs to be opened during radical pelvic operations, such as radical hysterectomy, pelvic lymphadenectomy and exenterative procedures, or some bladder suspension operations. However, it is used during laparoscopic hysterectomy to identify and free the lateral umbilical ligament or obliterated hypogastric artery (see below).

Surgical anatomy of the ureter

The ureters vary between 25 and 30 cm in length, depending on the height of the individual, and its two components (abdominal and pelvic) are approximately equal in length. The ureters pass along the anterior surface of the psoas muscles to the pelvic inlet; they are covered by the colon on either side, and are crossed anteriorly by the left and right colic arteries in the bowel mesentery. In their abdominal course, the ureters lie lateral to the ovarian vessels, but they enter the pelvis by crossing underneath the infundibulopelvic ligaments, and actually lie medial to the infundibulopelvic ligaments at the pelvic brim (Fig. 10.5). Upon crossing the pelvic brim, the ureters descend in the pelvis in a connective-tissue sheath, which is attached to the medial leaf of the broad ligament and the pelvic side-wall and lies just above the internal iliac arteries. At the level of the ischial spine, the ureters run forward and medially in the base of the broad ligament to enter the cardinal ligament. They pass under the uterine arteries approximately 1.5 cm lateral to the internal cervical os (Fig. 10.6). The left ureter is usually closer to the cervix than the right. The ureters then turn abruptly medially to enter the bladder, passing over the anterior vaginal fornices as they do so. The terminal 1–2 cm of the ureter is called the genu or knee of the ureter.

These anatomical relationships have three important practical consequences:

1 *Because the ureter is intimately related to the infundibulopelvic ligament*, it can be damaged during ligation and division of the ligament. The risk

* The reader may find that, in some anatomy texts, the lateral umbilical ligament is, confusingly enough, called the *medial* umbilical ligament. Those, such as Netter, who use this bizarre nomenclature for these lateral structures refer to the urachus as the *median* umbilical ligament, whereas we would call the urachus the *medial* umbilical ligament.

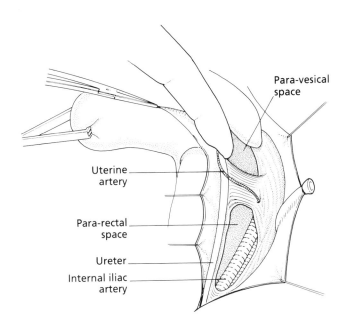

Fig. 10.4 The paravesical space has been developed bluntly. The obliterated hypogastric artery lies against the dissecting finger.

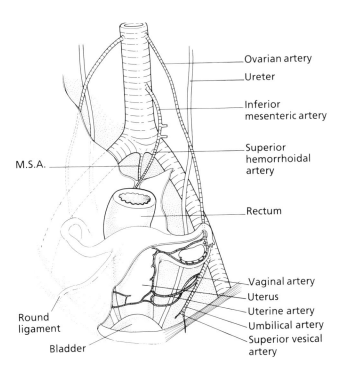

Fig. 10.5 The anatomical relations of the abdominal and pelvic ureter. The ureter lies lateral to the ovarian vessels above the pelvis, but crosses under the infundibulopelvic ligament at the pelvic brim, and actually lies medial to it on the broad ligament. The infundibulopelvic ligament has to be retracted medially to expose the ureter at the pelvic brim.

of ureteric injury increases the closer the ligament is divided to the pelvic brim.

2 *Because the ureter lies medial to the infundibulopelvic ligament at the pelvic brim*, the ligament has to be pulled medially to expose the ureter laparoscopically at the pelvic brim.

3 *Because of its proximity to the cervix at the level of the cardinal ligament*, the ureter is prone to injury during division of the cardinal

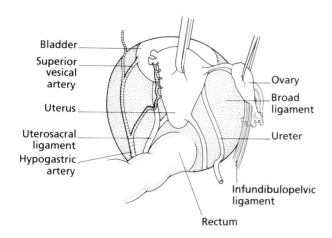

Fig. 10.6 The ureter is crossed by the uterine artery about 1.5–2 cm from the cervix, and it is tethered to the undersurface of the artery by the areolar tissue, which must be separated to allow the ureter to be displaced laterally. On the right, the ureter can be seen through the back of the broad ligament by anteflexing the uterus.

ligament, and also during division of the uterine artery, if the artery is divided low where it lies on top of the cardinal ligament.

When an open approach is used, dissection of the retroperitoneum and ureters is seldom necessary if hysterectomy or adnexal surgery is being carried out for benign pathology. The reasons are twofold. First, the ureters can be palpated in the broad ligament after the infundibulopelvic ligaments or adnexa are clamped to ensure that they have not been included in the clamps. Second, the technique used in a simple hysterectomy to clamp the uterine arteries, the parametria and the cardinal ligaments, ensures that only tissue directly adjacent to the cervix, and therefore medial to the ureter, is included in the clamps. The technique entails clamping the uterine arteries high on the uterus, where they lie medial to the ureter, and then placing all subsequent clamps medial to the uterine pedicle in such a way that the cervix is partly included in each 'bite' and then slowly allowed to escape from the clamps as their jaws are closed. After the cardinal ligament is clamped, the ureter can also be palpated below the clamp prior to division of the tissues. (A similar technique for clamp placement but in reverse order safeguards the ureter during vaginal hysterectomy.)

None of these options are available when a laparoscopic approach is used. It is relatively easy to visualize the ureter in the broad ligament laparoscopically, and the uterine arteries can be coagulated or sutured high on the uterus, but the strategies used to safeguard the ureters as the parametria and cardinal ligaments are clamped during an abdominal or vaginal hysterectomy cannot be employed with a laparoscopic approach. The ureters lie 1–2 cm from the cervix and, unless they are displaced laterally away from the cervix, they can be damaged by lateral spread of the current, if the cardinal ligaments are coagulated with bipolar diathermy prior to division, or crushed, if the cardinal ligaments are stapled. Stapling devices such as Endo GIA (US Surgical Corp., Norwalk, CT) are wider than clamps (1.1 cm) and their jaws do not open wide enough for the device to be placed in the same way as a clamp when the cardinal ligaments are stapled. Consequently, the Endo GIA can never be placed as close to the cervix as a clamp.

The corollary is that, if the cardinal and uterosacral ligaments have to be divided laparoscopically rather than vaginally, the ureters must be not only identified but actually displaced further away from the cervix than where they naturally lie. In practice, this means that they have to be freed from the under-surface of the uterine arteries to which they are tethered by areolar tissue. Once this is done and the uterine arteries are divided, the ureters can be pushed away from the cervix and the cardinal and uterosacral ligaments safely divided.

Laparoscopic identification of the ureter

The ureter can be identified laparoscopically and dissected free of surrounding tissues in one of three ways, which may be called the medial, superior and lateral approaches.

The medial approach

The medial approach to the ureter is the simplest and most commonly used, but it is the least versatile. It consists of sharply anteflexing the uterus to enable the ureter to be visualized through the peritoneum of the broad ligament in its natural position on the pelvic side-wall (see Fig. 10.6). The peritoneum immediately above the ureter is then incised to create a 'window' in the peritoneum, which allows the infundibulo-pelvic ligament or adnexal pedicle to be safely divided. The peritoneal incision must be very superficial, otherwise the iliac vessels can be injured. The limitations of this approach are that it cannot be used if pelvic pathology obscures the broad ligament, and that it does not allow proper development of the pararectal space. Identification of the ureter on the medial leaf of the broad ligament will also not facilitate division of the cardinal ligament, for this requires freeing of the ureter from the uterine artery above and lateral displacement of the ureter.

The superior approach

The superior approach to ureteric identification is also occasionally employed during laparotomy, when the retroperitoneal spaces have been obliterated by prior extraperitoneal surgery. The technique entails identifying the ureter above the pelvic brim, and then tracing it into the pelvis along the medial leaf of the broad ligament. When this is done laparoscopically, a key manoeuvre is to pull the infundibulopelvic ligament medially to expose the underlying ureter; on the left side, the congenital adhesions of the sigmoid colon sometimes have to be divided. Once the ureter has been identified and freed superiorly, it is then progressively reflected off the medial leaf of the broad ligament until the uterine vessels are reached. Reich [1, 2] uses this approach on the left side (and the medial approach on the right), but the dissection tends to be time-consuming and laborious because the broad ligament becomes increasingly lax as the dissection proceeds. Moreover, extensive mobilization of that part of the ureter which lies more than a few centimetres proximal to the uterine arteries, and which makes up most of the dissection, serves little useful purpose unless a radical hysterectomy is being performed, for it in no way facilitates subsequent division of the uterine arteries or cardinal ligaments.

The lateral approach

The lateral approach to the ureter is the one used by pelvic surgeons during laparotomy, and consists of opening the pararectal space as previously described. I have used the lateral approach to laparoscopic ureteric dissection during three laparoscopically assisted radical vaginal hysterectomies and bilateral pelvic lymphadenectomies, and 21 simple laparoscopic hysterectomies, three of which were combined with bilateral pelvic lymphadenectomy. The dissection proved to be tedious and difficult because the pararectal spaces cannot easily be developed laparoscopically in the same way as during a laparotomy. First, the internal iliac artery is buried in areolar tissues and cannot be immediately visualized after opening the broad ligament, and obviously cannot be palpated (see Fig. 10.2). Second, the precise level (in a cephalad–caudad sense) at which to begin dissecting the pararectal space is also not at first obvious, and troublesome bleeding can occur if the dissection is begun over the cardinal ligament rather than proximal to it. Finally, with each successive step of the dissection, that is, division of the round ligament, opening of the broad ligament, separation of the areolar tissues, the tissues become progressively more slack and difficult to work with.

A technique was therefore developed specifically to overcome these difficulties, which makes use of two strategies [3]. First, the round ligaments are divided late in the course of the dissection rather than at the beginning of it, which allows them to provide some counter-traction on the broad ligament when the uterus is deviated to the contralateral side. Second, the obliterated hypogastric arteries (lateral umbilical ligaments) are used to identify the origin of the uterine arteries, which are then used as landmarks for the pararectal spaces and ureters.

A laparoscopic technique for identifying the ureter: the modified lateral approach

The obliterated hypogastric arteries are a continuation of the internal iliac arteries (or, more properly, their anterior divisions); they sweep upwards on either side of the bladder, cross the superior pubic rami and run beneath the peritoneum of the anterior abdominal wall to the umbilicus. These structures are easily identified laparoscopically as prominent peritoneal folds that hang laterally on either side of the anterior abdominal wall; they are also relatively fixed and therefore easily dissected free of the bladder and surrounding areolar tissues. Once freed, each obliterated hypogastric artery can easily be traced to where it (or what is now more properly called the superior vesicle artery) is joined by the uterine artery to form the internal iliac artery (see Fig. 10.5).

The first step in the dissection is to delineate the triangle of the pelvic side-wall by displacing the uterus to the contralateral side. The base of this triangle is formed by the round ligament, the lateral border by the external iliac artery, the medial border by the infundibulopelvic ligament, and the apex by where the infundibulopelvic ligament crosses the common iliac artery (Fig. 10.7). The peritoneum in the middle of the triangle is incised with the unopened tips of the endoshears (US Surgical Corp., Norwalk, CT), using a monopolar cutting current, and the broad ligament is opened by bluntly separating the extraperitoneal areolar tissues (Fig. 10.8). Even tiny vessels should be coagulated because the slightest amount of bleeding can stain the extraperitoneal areolar tissues and obscure a view of the underlying structures. The peritoneal incision is extended towards the apex of the pelvic side-wall triangle, and the infundibulopelvic ligament is pulled medially with grasping forceps to expose the ureter at the pelvic brim, where it crosses the common or external iliac artery (Fig. 10.9). On the left side the apex of the triangle is often covered by the sigmoid colon, which has then to be first mobilized by dividing the adhesions that tether it to the pelvic brim.

After the pelvic side-wall triangle and broad ligament have been

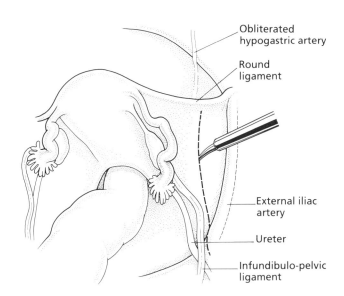

Obliterated hypogastric artery

Round ligament

External iliac artery

Ureter

Infundibulo-pelvic ligament

Fig. 10.7 The uterus has been deviated to the left to delineate the right pelvic side-wall triangle, and the peritoneum in the middle of the triangle is incised.

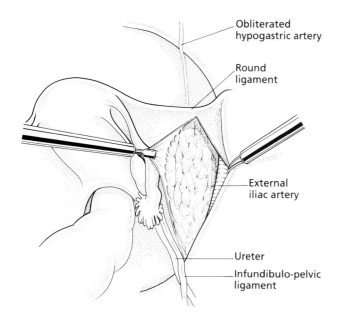

Fig. 10.8 After incising the peritoneum, the leaves of the broad ligament are separated by blunt dissection.

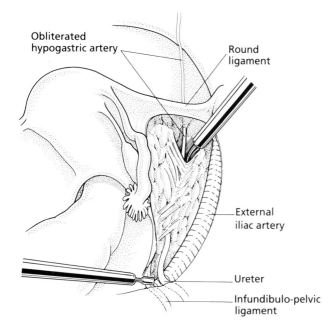

Fig. 10.9 The obliterated hypogastric artery is identified extraperitoneally by blunt dissection of the retroperitoneal areolar tissues.

opened, the dissection is carried bluntly underneath and caudad to the round ligament, which is *not* divided at this time, until the obliterated hypogastric artery is identified extraperitoneally. This is easily done because the obliterated hypogastric artery is a relatively fixed structure lying just medial to the lower portion of the external iliac artery and vein (see Fig. 10.9). If any difficulty is encountered, the artery can be traced proximally from where it hangs from the anterior abdominal wall and identified extraperitoneally. Identification is further facilitated by moving the intraperitoneal part of the ligament back and forth and observing the corresponding movements in the extraperitoneal portion of the ligament.

Using blunt dissection, the areolar tissue lateral to the obliterated hypogastric artery is separated to open the paravesical space. If a radical hysterectomy or pelvic lymphadenectomy is to be performed, this space is opened down to the levator floor; otherwise the dissection is intended only to delineate the lateral border of the artery (Fig. 10.10). The medial border of the artery is then freed (Fig. 10.11), and the artery traced proximally to where it is joined by the uterine artery to form the internal iliac artery (Fig. 10.12).

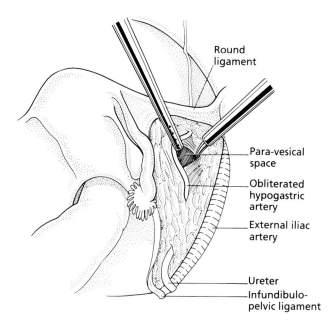

Fig. 10.10 The paravesical space is opened lateral to the obliterated hypogastric artery.

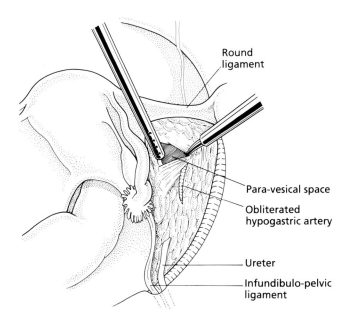

Fig. 10.11 The medial border of the obliterated hypogastric artery is freed from the bladder.

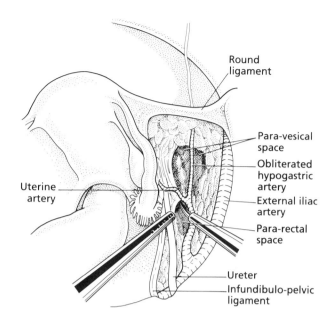

Fig. 10.12 The obliterated hypogastric artery is traced proximally to where it is joined by the uterine artery. The pararectal space is developed by blunt dissection proximal and medial to the uterine artery, the ureter is identified on the medial border of the pararectal space and the uterine artery is traced down to where it crosses the ureter.

The uterine arteries mark the top of the cardinal ligaments, which form the caudad limit of the pararectal spaces. Therefore, the uterine arteries provide a useful landmark of where to open the pararectal spaces, and help to avoid the unnecessary bleeding which can result if the dissection is started either too proximally or too distally. The pararectal spaces are developed by blunt dissection just proximal and medial to the uterine arteries; once the pararectal space has been opened, the ureter on that side is easily identified for it forms the medial border of the pararectal space (see Fig. 10.12).

The pararectal space is developed to the extent needed for the operation being performed — as far as the levator floor if the operation is a radical hysterectomy, or sufficiently to identify the ureter if a simple hysterectomy is to be performed. Fine areolar tissue tethers the ureter to the under-surface of the uterine artery, and this is most easily separated bluntly by introducing and spreading the jaws of a mixter clamp (Jarit Inc., Hawthorne, NY) underneath the artery. For a simple hysterectomy the uterine artery should be divided above or medial to the ureter, after which the ureter can be pushed laterally to allow the cardinal ligament to be safely divided. Before doing so, however, the distal part of the ureter is peeled off the uterosacral ligament, and each ligament divided close to its attachment to the cervix.

After performing several pelvic side-wall dissections, both with and without ureteric stents, I have become convinced that the dissection is facilitated by having stents in place, even though I have never found stents to be the slightest bit useful during laparotomy and never use them for open cases. The stents make the ureters much more prominent and rigid, and therefore easier to see and dissect against, and they prevent the ureters from falling out of view into the depths of the pelvis after they are freed. The purpose of the stents is *not* to allow the ureters to be 'felt' endoscopically. The technique of placing ureteric stents is extremely straightforward and can be quickly mastered by any gynaecologist trained in cystoscopy. Stents also provide a safeguard against unrecognized ureteric injury.

Summary and conclusions

Techniques for removing the uterus laparoscopically and the nomenclature for these procedures are discussed at length in other chapters of this book. A central and recurring question will be whether or not the ureters need to be dissected free of their surrounding tissues. It is important at the outset to distinguish between identifying the ureter and actually dissecting it free, although admittedly it is sometimes necessary to free the ureter to be able to see it laparoscopically if there are extensive pelvic adhesions or the tissues have become excessively bloodstained. The anatomical relations of the ureter should make it obvious that the position of the ureter during hysterectomy must be known before any of the pedicles are divided. However, the ureter only needs to be dissected free of the surrounding tissues if it has to be actually displaced from its natural position to enable some step of the operation to be safely performed. From the anatomical relations of the ureter it should again be evident that this is only required if the cardinal and, to a lesser extent, the uterosacral ligaments are to be divided laparoscopically.

The inability to place tissues on sufficient tension is a major encumberance during laparoscopic pelvic surgery and renders pelvic side-wall dissection and ureteric identification particularly difficult. A technique has been developed specifically to overcome these difficulties, which relies on the anatomical relations of the obliterated hypogastric artery. The sequence in which the dissection is carried out is also important in order to preserve the natural tension in the tissues for as long as possible. Although the anatomy of the pelvic vasculature is subject to considerable variation, there is a constant relationship between the obliterated hypogastric and the uterine arteries. The level at which the uterine artery is given off varies somewhat, and the uterine artery may sometimes divide into two branches, one below and one above the ureter, but these minor differences do not in any way affect or interfere with the basic strategy and dissection. In my experience, the lateral umbilical ligaments were no less prominent or more difficult to identify in patients weighing over 200 pounds, or in those who had either extensive pelvic adhesions obliterating the cul-de-sac or previous major pelvic surgery, or both.

References

1 Reich H. Laparoscopic hysterectomy. *Surg Laparoscopy Endoscopy* 1992; **2**: 85–88.
2 Reich H. Pelvic sidewall dissection. *Clin Obstet Gynecol* 1991; **34** (2): 412–422.
3 Kadar N. A laparoscopic technique for dissecting the pelvic retroperitoneum and identifying the ureters. *Am J Obstet Gynecol* (submitted for publication).

11: Anaesthesia for Gynaecological Endoscopic Surgery

Minimally invasive surgery challenges anaesthetists as much as it challenges gynaecologists and surgeons and it is important that new anaesthetic approaches are developed to ensure that these 'minimally invasive' techniques are truly safe and associated with minimal complications and rapid recovery. Recent improvements in anaesthetic techniques for laparoscopic procedures have increased the patient acceptance and the medical acceptability of short-stay laparoscopic surgery.

Anaesthetic considerations

The choice of optimum anaesthetic technique can be made more rational if the physiological changes of laparoscopy are understood. Most laparoscopic procedures are performed with the patient positioned in both a lithotomy and a steep Trendelenberg (15–30°) position. In addition, the abdomen is distended with gas under pressure. The combined effect of this position and the pneumatoperitoneum is to cause adverse physiological changes, particularly in the respiratory and cardiovascular systems. With the abdominal contents pushed cephalad, there is splinting of the diaphragm with impairment of ventilation and respiratory mechanics. There are observed decreases in lung compliance, vital capacity and functional residual capacity, coupled with an increase in the pulmonary blood volume. Pulmonary compliance is reduced and there is an increase in ventilation/perfusion mismatch as a result of basal compression and the redistribution of hydrostatic forces. The above effects can be demonstrated in healthy volunteers and are exaggerated by insufflation of gases and further compounded by the effects of anaesthesia. Obese patients and those with cardiovascular disease are particularly vulnerable to these changes and are prone to postoperative atelectasis and pneumonia, especially when the operative procedure is prolonged.

The most commonly used insufflation gas is carbon dioxide. Much of this is absorbed from the peritoneal cavity and this absorption appears to increase after deflation of the abdomen. This increased absorption after deflation suggests that absorption is increased when the abdominal pressure is reduced. This absorption of CO_2 results in a metabolic and respiratory acidosis with an increased respiratory rate. The acidosis may lead to cardiac arrhythmias, especially if halothane is used to supplement the anaesthesia. There is, however, no significant change in the partial pressure of oxygen in the arterial blood, due to a decreased alveolar-to-arterial pressure gradient caused by the raised cardiac output which occurs during the postural physiological changes in the Trendelenberg position (Table 11.1).

Other complications of the pneumatoperitoneum include venous gas embolism. This was much more common when the less soluble gas, nitrous oxide, was used. The incidence of gas embolism has been reduced with the regular use of carbon dioxide because it is much more soluble. Nitrous oxide is also more diffusible and can enter the bowel, with consequent distension and impairment of vision during laparoscopy. Mediastinal and abdominal-wall emphysema may also occur, particularly if the intra-abdominal pressure is grossly elevated during insufflation.

Table 11.1 Anaesthetic complications of laparoscopy

Hypercarbia
Acid–base disturbance
Hypoxia
Cardiac arrhythmias
Hypotension
Gas embolism
Pneumothorax/pneumomediastinum
Pulmonary aspiration

Anaesthetic technique

The choice of anaesthetic in this as in all other types of surgery is determined by the condition of the patient, the extent of the surgery, the personal preference of the anaesthetist and the facilities available. Laparoscopy can be performed under general, regional or local anaesthesia. Advanced laparoscopic techniques, however, are often prolonged and, taking into account the previously mentioned physiological effects, general anaesthesia with controlled ventilation is the treatment of choice. Advantages include airway protection, optimum operating conditions and analgesia. Controlled ventilation minimizes or may even reverse the physiological changes that result from the effects of position and the pneumatoperitoneum. In our opinion, spontaneous ventilation has no place in prolonged laparoscopic procedures as it does not provide optimum operating or physiological conditions. Patients are selected for elective day surgery on: (i) the type of procedure to be performed; and (ii) the ASA status of the patient (Table 11.2). Patients in ASA categories 1 and 2 may be suitable for day-case stay but those in other groups will need to be admitted for preoperative assessment and postoperative observation, whatever degree of surgery is performed.

Table 11.2 ASA physical status scale

Class 1 A normal healthy individual
Class 2 A patient with mild systemic disease
Class 3 A patient with a severe but not incapacitating illness
Class 4 A patient with incapacitating systemic disease that is a constant threat to life
Class 5 A moribund patient not expected to live 24 hours with or without surgery

Premedication

The purpose of premedication is to reduce anxiety and anaesthetic problems. Much can be done, however, with adequate explanation, reassurance and counselling by all the staff. The value of a purpose-designed unit specializing in short-stay surgery, appropriately staffed by experienced medical and nursing staff able to give appropriate advice, cannot be overestimated. If anxiety persists, a short-acting benzodiazepine such as temazepam is often adequate (Table 11.3).

Table 11.3 Anaesthetic techniques

Sleep
Analgesia
Muscle relaxation
Monitoring

Anaesthetic

The induction agent chosen is usually an ultra-short-acting barbiturate such as thiopentone or, with increasing frequency, the phenol derivative, propofol (Diprivan, ICI, Cheshire). Propofol has the major advantage that it allows a much more rapid awakening and better recovery.

Muscle relaxation is required and is best produced with a short-acting agent such as vecuronium or atracurium, which are given in bolus incremental doses during the procedure without running risks of accumulation if the procedure should be prolonged. With this protocol, a cuffed endotracheal tube should always be used to protect the particularly vulnerable airway and to facilitate controlled ventilation.

Maintenance of the anaesthetic may be provided with either inhalation or intravenous agents. Halothane, enflurane and isoflurane have all been used successfully. Halothane, however, predisposes to cardiac arrhythmias in the presence of hypercarbia, and isoflurane is the most expensive of these agents. Analgesia during the procedure can safely be provided with short-acting opiates such as fentanyl or alfentanyl. These short-acting opiates are less likely to cause respiratory depression in the postoperative period.

Adequate monitoring is essential to detect any potential complication that may occur. The minimal monitoring required for laparoscopy should include continuous electrocardiography to detect cardiac arrhythmias and ischaemia, non-invasive blood-pressure, pulse oximetry to measure oxygen saturation and, most essentially, capnography to detect breath changes in the end-tidal CO_2 tension. With this last piece of information, the ventilation can be altered to control the CO_2 tension within normal limits.

Postoperative analgesia

In spite of these procedures being 'minimally invasive', there is often significant postoperative pain following laparoscopy. Patients may complain of both abdominal pain and sometimes quite distressing shoulder-tip pain. This may be due to pain referred from diaphragmatic irritation due to fluid and blood in the peritoneal cavity. The other possible cause is the formation of carbonic acid, from the mixing of CO_2 and water, which then irritates the peritoneal surfaces. In the immediate postoperative period, opiates remain the mainstay of severe pain relief, followed by simple oral analgesics such as paracetamol. The non-steroidal anti-inflammatory agents are also becoming popular.

Analgesic techniques, like their surgical counterparts, are improving all the time. We have had very encouraging results from the use of patient-controlled analgesia in patients who have had prolonged laparoscopic procedures.

Regional anaesthesia

Regional anaesthesia has been successfully used for laparoscopy, particularly in ill patients in whom general anaesthesia is contraindicated. Local infiltrations are inadequate and epidurals may result in complications. A regional block must be high and extend up to T_4 to prevent diaphragmatic discomfort. A block at this level may also result in hypotension and ventilatory dysfunction due to the motor blockade of the intercostal muscles. We do not recommend regional anaesthetic techniques for prolonged laparoscopic procedures.

Summary

We have tried in this chapter to provide an overview of the problems that prolonged laparoscopic surgery produces for the anaesthetist. We have described the procedures we think are most suitable for this type of surgery. There is, however, no substitute for continuing rapport between the surgeon and the anaesthetist to ensure continued safe and judicious patient management.

12: Nursing Problems Associated with Laparoscopic Surgery

In the operating room (OR)

The theatre nurse's role has changed dramatically with the introduction of advanced laparoscopic surgery. The nurse is confronted with new challenges and added responsibilities. She/He must learn to work with, and care for, electronic and laser instrumentation and must be capable of keeping this equipment in a state of instant readiness. Without a committed and informed support team, the introduction of new techniques will not be successful and surgeon and nurses must share a common enthusiasm for these exciting new procedures.

I believe that the use of so much new equipment and so many novel techniques makes the endoscopic surgical nurse a subspeciality of theatre nursing as valid as, say, orthopaedic or plastic surgery. It is important that our medical staff and our nursing peers recognize this new speciality, for it is only with such recognition that adequate training and educational support will be given to the whole team.

The introduction of laser technology into the operating room provokes perhaps the greatest change in approach and procedures. With lasers, as with all equipment, it is important to ensure an adequate safety policy. A class IV laser is a high-powered laser which emits radiation at levels that can produce harmful effects from direct and reflected radiation. The eyes are the most vulnerable area and care must be taken to ensure adequate protection. A laser protection supervisor is necessary to establish and ensure that laser safety policy is implemented and to provide ongoing safety education and training for all staff who work in the vicinity of class IV lasers.

A laser safety committee, with representatives from all interested specialities, should be established to ensure that the agreed safety policies are implemented. A medical physicist or similarly qualified person should be appointed as a laser protection adviser, who will prepare the local safety policies and procedures. Once agreed, these should be prominently displayed outside the laser area so that all personnel working near the area are aware of the hazards associated with lasers. These should be confined to specifically designated laser areas. These laser areas should have removable warning signs which should indicate the following:

1 Eye protection must be worn when the laser is activated.
2 The warning laser triangle should be displayed.
3 The extent of the restricted area.
4 A warning to beware of direct and scattered laser beams.

There should be a separate sign for each laser class and wavelength, displaying the maximum wattage output of the particular laser in use. Appropriate eye protection from the laser should also be available at every entrance for anyone who must enter the restricted area when the warning signs are illuminated. All glass windows must be covered with opaque material and a warning sign should be illuminated when the laser is in the 'ready mode'.

When the surgeon requests the laser to be made ready, the laser operator must ensure that all staff and the patient are wearing adequate eye protection and the warning signs are illuminated before clearly repeating the 'laser ready' instruction and confirming the power setting e.g. '10 watts'. At the end of the procedure, the request of the surgeon for 'laser off' is confirmed by the response 'stand-by'. The laser operator should have no other responsibilities during the procedure and should stay with the laser when it is in the ready mode. If it is necessary for her/him to leave, the laser must be switched to stand-by.

A laser can be an electrical hazard and it is important that fluids should not be placed on top of the laser. Care must be taken to ensure that the laser is only fired when the beam is directed at the intended treatment site, to avoid any fire risk. A container of saline should be readily available and a CO_2 fire-extinguisher should be near by. Drapes can be a fire hazard. Single-use disposable drapes are designed to be water-repellent and, if ignited, fluid used to douse the flames may roll away and not reach the seat of the fire. Inflammable skin-preparation solutions should not be used but, if their use is unavoidable, the area prepared should be carefully dried prior to draping.

A register of authorized laser users (medical) and laser operators (nursing) must be kept and updated as necessary. Access to the laser should be restricted to registered users.

To those unused to working with lasers, the duties listed above may sound formidable but in practice similar precautions and duties are required for most of the other items of equipment required for advanced laparoscopic surgery. It is the nursing staff's responsibility to ensure that all the electronic equipment and the more conventional surgical instruments are available, cleaned and functional before the operating session begins. Each item of equipment should be tested. A blown fuse, failed bulb or loose wire can easily be detected and rectified prior to the patient being anaesthetized. Problems not detected until later may delay the operation or even be a hazard for the patient.

The video unit should be switched on and checked. The monitor, slave monitor, light source, camera cables, camera control unit and video-recorder should all be inspected. Particular care should be taken to ensure that all the many connections are sound and the switches correctly set. Adequate supplies of video-tape, spare batteries and camera films should be available. The endocamera lens should be clean, dry and polished. The smallest amount of moisture in the lens system may cause troublesome fogging. We no longer sterilize the camera by soaking it in glutaraldehyde solution. This not only avoids problems with fogging but also avoids the ever-present danger of seepage of the solution into the camera with consequent damage. We find it adequate to clean the camera with a sterile moist towel and wipe the surface and then wrap the camera body in an alco-wipe until ready for use. After use, the camera and cable should be thoroughly washed in warm soapy water, dried and stored in a foam-lined box with the lens covers removed. A sachet of desiccant in the box will keep the camera moisture-free.

CO_2 insufflator

The cylinder of CO_2 needs to be turned on, the gas level checked and the internal reservoir, if present, filled ready for connection to the patient. Most newer insufflators require special sets of disposable silicone tubing with appropriate connectors, all of which should be sterile. It is necessary to periodically check the volume of CO_2 remaining in the main cylinder, particularly during prolonged procedures, and spare cylinders must be readily available for speedy interchange when necessary.

Irrigation unit

An adequate supply of normal saline or Ringer's lactate bottles must be available at the correct temperature. Many irrigating units are powered by pressurized CO_2 and the cylinders must again be full at the start of a major procedure, with spares available. Some surgeons prefer heparin to be added to the irrigation fluid, and this should be added, when appropriate, to the fluid.

Suction unit

A suitable suction system, with appropriate tubing and connectors and collecting vessels, must also be assembled and checked.

All this equipment must be carefully arranged to reduce clutter, facilitate access to the patient and ensure the monitors are in the optimum positions for the surgeon and the staff. Tower trolleys are particularly helpful in this regard, and a suggested arrangement has been described in Chapter 3.

Operative instruments

All endoscopic instruments should be cleaned by the theatre team who are responsible for them. Reusable laparoscopic cannulae with trumpet valves should be dismantled for cleaning. The trumpet valve in this type of cannula is made of brass and becomes tarnished with use. Cleaning with metal polish and lubricating with instrument oil after every use ensures a smooth action. Gas taps require similar attention to prevent stiffness.

Grasping forceps, suction probes and morcellators all require dismantling after use for proper cleaning. A high-pressure water-gun is very helpful for flushing narrow channels free of trapped debris. Trocar points should be examined for sharpness. Sealing caps frequently split; they should be examined and defective ones replaced. Some endoscopic instruments are quite complex to strip down and reassemble; this is especially true of the morcellator, which must be completely dismantled after every use for thorough cleaning and maintenance. When in a satisfactory condition, the instruments should be sent for packing and autoclaving. When possible, instruments should be autoclaved with the jaws open to relieve tension on the closure mechanism.

To avoid risk of damage to delicate and heat-sensitive components, telescopes and light cables should be immersed in a chemical sterilization fluid such as glutaraldehyde. Thorough cleaning before immersion is essential, as glutaraldehyde will 'fix' blood and proteins. The advantage of glutaraldehyde is that it is active over a wide range of bacteria and organisms, including TB, spores and viruses (including HIV), and yet it does not damage rubber, metal, plastic or lens cement. Thorough rinsing is essential because of the toxic, irritant properties of the solution. Immersion times should be as recommended by the manufacturers. Glutaraldehyde is a hazardous substance to work with as it is irritant to the eyes, skin and lungs. Eye protection should be worn and it should only be used in adequately ventilated areas. It must be stored in dedicated immersion tanks with tight-fitting lids.

Storage of endoscopic instruments can be a problem as they are numerous and delicate and must be instantly available. We have found the RIWO trolley (Richard Wolfe Ltd) to be particularly useful for this purpose. It has six trays for storage, which, when foam-lined and 'shallow cut', provide safe storage for telescopes. Two drawers provide storage for many different sealing caps, washers and spare parts. The top shelf has two tanks with fume-tight lids for glutaraldehyde, with timers built into the lids for checking immersion times.

All other, less delicate instruments should be autoclaved. With a busy schedule, it is important to ensure that there are sufficient instruments available to cover the time out of the OR and this must be considered when deciding on the quantity of instruments to be purchased. Theatre nurses should be consulted by the medical staff for an evaluation of the quality, durability and ease of cleaning and reassembly of equipment used. All instruments purchased should be user-friendly. Repair and replacement services offered by different manufacturers vary greatly and reputations should be considered when making any purchase.

Drapes

A draping system for advanced laparoscopy procedures can be troublesome if towels constantly come adrift and do not adequately cover the patient. Specifically designed disposable systems are available and we have found the Baxter health-care convertor range particularly suitable. The laparoscopic pack consists of two leggings and a large abdominal sheet with a triangular cut-out with adhesive edges which adhere to the patient's abdomen in the correct position, thus eliminating slipping. There is an extra-absorbent area around the cut-out to prevent spillage of blood and irrigating fluids. There are also loops adjacent to the operating sites through which the optic cables and fluid and gas lines can be passed. These lines are thereby securely held in the correct position and yet still able to run free. There is also a second, oblong cut-out area for the perineum. A novel feature of this system is the paper flap, which can be used to initially cover the abdominal area whilst the preliminary catheterization and uterine manipulations are being performed and which can then be pivoted to cover the perineum for the major part of the laparoscopic surgery.

Fibre light cables

Fibre light cables should be checked before use for broken fibres. These can be seen as black spots when the fibre is lit. Such damage causes a sharp reduction in the amount of light transmitted. A cable should be replaced when 25% of the fibres are damaged. For optimum light transmission, the fibre bundle of the cable should be bigger than the fibre bundle of the telescope. A 2.5-mm telescope requires 3.5-mm light cable, etc. The fibre cables should be carefully stored, loosely coiled and not kinked.

Surrounded by all this 'high-tech' equipment, the nurse and all the theatre team must not forget that under the drapes is a patient. Even the title 'minimally invasive surgery' can be misleading. The patients are often undergoing major surgical procedures and require at least as high a level of nursing care and skills as would be required with traditional open surgery. These procedures are often very time-consuming and prolonged. When complications such as haemorrhage or ruptured viscera occur, the surgeon requires immediate skilled and effective help. If conversion to laparotomy is required, considerable previous experience and skills in open surgery will also be required.

Positioning of the patient

This is also usually a nursing procedure. Patients undergoing laparoscopic procedures are often in our care for long periods of time. The position on the table must be as safe and as comfortable as possible. The position chosen must also give as much access as possible and these two priorities are often in conflict. The patient will be in the lithotomy position and the leg supports should be well padded and carefully placed to avoid pressure on nerves and vessels in the legs. The sacrum should be supported and not allowed to overhang the table. It must, however, be placed as close as possible to the edge to allow maximum room for uterine manipulation. The legs should be abducted as far as comfortably possible to maximize space between the legs for vaginal surgery. At the same time, they should be maintained in a 'low' lithotomy position with the hips flexed at an angle of 145° to the abdomen to maximize the space available for laparoscopic manoeuvres. To achieve this the lithotomy poles should be secured at this angle.

The patient's arms should be placed by her side and the patient then placed in a steep Trendelenberg, the degree of which will be adjusted during the operation. The patient's eyes are protected with moistened gauze swabs placed over the eyelids and, if lasers are to be used, protective goggles are then applied.

The endoscopic theatre nurse must act as the patient's advocate during the period she is in surgery. When treating patients in this specialized way, patient preoperative and postoperative care must be just as specialized, and close links between ward, out-patient and theatre staff must be maintained. The other groups should be encouraged to come to theatre and observe the new procedures at first hand.

As this section describes, advanced, laparoscopic surgery poses many new challenges for theatre nurses. They urgently require information, education and communication. Nurse training and education is much neglected and yet essential for a successful endoscopic surgical programme. The scrub nurse assisting the surgeon needs to develop precise hand–eye co-ordination and a refined sense of depth perception. These skills are not inherent and need to be taught for this role to be filled with confidence. Nursing courses, workshops and journals on endoscopic surgical techniques are required. Nurses need training, support, information and the opportunity to share their experiences with their colleagues to enable them to offer their patients the highest possible standards.

On the ward

The introduction of advanced laparoscopic techniques has had a profound effect on the nursing activities in our gynaecological wards. When a patient undergoes conventional abdominal or vaginal hysterectomy, she is inevitably admitted to the unit the day before and stays between 5 and 8 days after the procedure. This prolonged in-patient stay obviously limits the number of patients who can be so treated. The first and most immediate effect of minimally invasive endoscopic surgery is to greatly reduce the in-patient stay and consequently greatly increase the number of bed-days available. This almost inevitably also results in an increase in the number of patients who can be treated from a ward each week. It is important to ensure that the problems of rapid through-put are recognized and dealt with. The Audit Commission's first report on the UK Health Service noted 'that in order for day surgery to be used more extensively the problems of the effective management of short-stay patients must be resolved'.

Overcoming traditional views

Years of training and experience have accustomed nurses as well as their patients to expect a prolonged period of in-patient hospital care. At their encounter with minimally invasive surgery, therefore, nurses are initially reluctant to encourage early discharge for fear of the patient developing serious complications at home after being discharged too early! It is only with increasing experience and confidence in the procedures that the nurses are able to adopt the positive approach essential to implement these changes.

As the number of short-stay patients increases, the pressure on the nurses also increases. A particular area of strain is that, as the time between admission and going to theatre is short, there is little time to give the desired level of preoperative care. As the number of cases dealt with in such a manner increases, so does this strain. This procedure also means that patients who have developed medical problems or difficulties since their original consultation may have their operation cancelled because there is insufficient time to sort them out. The cancellation of a case, particularly if it could have been prevented, is distressing and inconvenient for the patient and a considerable waste of hospital resources.

This rushed environment provides little time for psychological preparation and satisfactory preoperative counselling. Patients are particularly vulnerable when they are admitted on the day of their operation. They have no time to adjust to their anxieties about the procedure. They are surrounded by entirely strange faces and then taken almost immediately to the operating room. These are very new procedures and patients' perceptions of what is involved vary widely.

We responded to this problem by introducing pre-clerking clinics, held the week before the patient is to be operated upon. At these clinics the patient is seen by members of both the medical and the nursing team who will care for her in hospital. The medical staff assess the patient for any changes in her gynaecological symptoms or her general health. Any necessary preoperative investigations are carried out. If there is a problem, the case can be postponed or altered, with enough time both to avoid any unnecessary distress for the patient and to send for a replacement case to fill the vacancy. The patient also has the opportunity to ask questions and identify any concerns at this visit.

The nurse's role is to complete the necessary documentation for her pre- and postoperative care and to allow time for discussion of problems. The admission details are repeated and advice such as attending with nil by mouth is reinforced. A particularly valuable aspect of this approach is that the patient meets some of the staff who will be caring for her during her hospital admission.

To summarize, pre-clerking clinics are a most cost-effective and socially effective method of preparing patients for short-stay surgery. They also reduce the activity in the wards at the time of surgery and ensure that the nursing staff are available for their primary caring roles at this time.

Safety aspects

The increased patient through-put and pace of admissions and discharges increase the risk of mistakes. It is essential to ensure that the highest possible standard of patient identification is maintained. A strict preoperative protocol must be followed and particular care taken to adhere to the local drug policies.

Postoperative problems

Patients who have undergone minimally invasive surgery have often had a major surgical procedure such as hysterectomy performed and yet are to be discharged within a short time. High-quality nursing care is essential to ensure that the patients are as fit as possible upon discharge. Regular recording of the vital signs is necessary following LH and LAVH to detect early signs of internal bleeding, bladder dysfunction or other complications associated with these procedures.

Analgesia

Ensuring adequate analgesia is important in short-stay surgery. Choosing the appropriate dose of the most suitable type of drug is essential. Too little pain relief will delay discharge and discredit the technique, while too much will cause drowsiness and nausea and again delay departure. Long-acting analgesics such as diclofenac suppositories can be effective. Many patients are helped to cope with mild or moderate postoperative discomfort with a 'take-home' pack of simple analgesics, which can both relieve the pain and reduce the level of anxiety.

For patients who have had laparoscopic-assisted hysterectomies, self-administered 'patient-controlled analgesia' systems have proved to be an effective means of giving excellent pain relief for the first 24 hours postoperatively. We restrict the use of this equipment to the first postoperative day because prolonged administration produces drowsiness and lack of mobility, which consequently delays the patient's return home. Following 24 hours of opiate analgesia, the patient is given adequate amounts of oral analgesia to maintain pain control whilst at the same time promoting early discharge. We use pain-score charts to help assess the effectiveness of the analgesia provided and to increase nursing and medical staff awareness of the patient's perception of her postoperative pain.

Nausea, if severe, can delay a patient's discharge and should be prevented if possible and vigorously controlled as quickly as possible if it occurs. An antiemetic is given in the operating theatre immediately after the operation has been completed. Reassurance that the nausea is transient is helpful and including a small supply of antiemetic in the 'take-home' pack is useful. Recently the introduction of long-acting skin-patch antiemetics has been found to be helpful.

Discharge home

Patients must be counselled about their anticipated early discharge home from the pre-clerking clinic onwards. While it may seem self-evident that all must welcome a short hospital stay, some patients have experienced conventional surgery and may anticipate and make arrangements for a longer stay. It is important that any discharge advice is given both verbally and in written form. Clear arrangements must be made about who to contact if they are anxious or concerned.

Staffing levels

The overall financial benefits of short-stay surgery are considerable. Shorter periods of in-patient hospital dependency do not, however, equate with fewer or less well-trained nursing staff. The increased turnover in fact usually results in the need for higher staffing levels. New working arrangements are necessary, with flexitime and other arrangements to ensure that the maximum number of staff are available at peak operating times. The employment of specific theatre-escort nurses is a means of ensuring rapid transfer of patients to and from theatre without depleting the wards of their skilled staff.

The introduction of this new approach to gynaecology has resulted in many changes of practice for nurses working on a short-stay gynaecology ward. It is essential that a dedicated and highly motivated team of nursing and medical staff join together to organize efficient and effective pre-clerking clinics, highly geared ward programmes and caring and yet flexible attitudes. Together we can help our patients to enjoy the benefits of minimally invasive surgery.

13: Results and Complications

The first laparoscopic hysterectomy was described in 1989 [1] and publications in the international literature on this subject are at present restricted to a few, single-case or very small number, preliminary type of reports. There has not been time to accumulate any long-term data on this procedure but it is not anticipated that the long-term results will differ in any significant way from those resulting from hysterectomy performed by more conventional routes.

Several centres have now, however, performed significant numbers of laparoscopic hysterectomies and the authors are particularly grateful to C.Y. Liu of Chattanooga and Alan Johns of Fort Worth for permission to present their unpublished results in this monograph. They have reported a total of 414 cases of laparoscopic hysterectomy and laparoscopic-assisted vaginal hysterectomy. In addition, we include the series of 36 cases reported by the Clermont-Ferrand group [2], as well as a series of 123 patients operated on by Harry Reich and a series of 75 patients operated upon by Padial *et al.* from Omaha, making a total of 648 cases for analysis.

The mean duration of these operations of varying extent and performed by surgeons of varying experience in advanced laparoscopic surgery at various stages of their learning curves was 117 min. The shortest operation took only 30 min and the longest some 6 hours 36 min. The mean time in hospital for patients undergoing laparoscopic hysterectomy was 1.83 days. 189 (92%) of 205 patients of Dr Liu were discharged within 24 hours of surgery (Tables 13.1 and 13.2).

Jeffrey Phipps, Michael John and Satish Nayak of Nuneaton, England, have recently completed an as yet unpublished, prospective, randomized

Table 13.1 Intraoperative details of laparoscopic hysterectomy cases

| Author | No. of cases | Duration of operation | | Length of hospital stay (days) |
		Average (min)	Range (min)	
Johns	199	79	30–240	2.46
Liu	215	114	45–340	1.21
Bruhat *et al.*	36	—	—	5.00
Reich	123	180	45–396	1.90
Padial *et al.*	75	121	—	2.37
	648 (total)	117 (mean)		2.07 (mean)

Table 13.2 Intraoperative complications of laparoscopic hysterectomy

Author	Urinary tract	Gastrointestinal	Postoperative pyrexia	Blood transfusion	Richter's hernia
John	3	—	2	—	—
Liu	4	2	1	1	1
Bruhat *et al.*	—	1	—	—	—
Reich	2	2	4	2	1
Padial *et al.*	—	—	8	—	—
Total	9	5	15	3	2

study comparing laparoscopic hysterectomy with abdominal hysterectomy. Their findings are summarized in Table 13.3.

In this interesting prospective study, laparoscopic hysterectomy was shown to be less painful, as judged by lower opiate requirements, and to result in an earlier discharge from hospital and earlier return to work. The operating time for laparoscopic hysterectomy was longer than that for abdominal hysterectomy. There were no operative or postoperative complications in either group in this small study.

In the larger studies the main intraoperative complication noted was bladder damage, which was encountered in five cases (a rate of 1.4%). Four of these were bladder fistulae, one of which occurred during vaginal dissection of the bladder. Two of the fistulae were successfully repaired laparoscopically at the time of the primary surgery. There were one case of damage to the ureter and one case of electrosurgical thermal damage to the sigmoid colon, which was repaired laparoscopically.

The principal postoperative complications were pyrexia (three cases), difficulty in voiding (three cases), a Richter's hernia and a case of subacute intestinal obstruction, which settled spontaneously. One patient required a postoperative blood transfusion. The overall complication rate in this composite group was only 4.2%.

The study of Phipps *et al.* is of particular interest, for it is the first prospective randomized study to compare laparoscopic hysterectomy with abdominal hysterectomy. The laparoscopic group required more than twice as long in theatre but stayed in hospital for only one-third

Table 13.3 Prospective study comparing abdominal and laparoscopic hysterectomy

Type of operation	No. of cases	Operating time (min)	Opiate required (mg)	Hospital stay (hours)	Return to work (weeks)
Abdominal	29	30	45	144	6
Laparoscopic	24	65	15	48	2

of the time (2 days vs. 6 days) and returned to work in 2 weeks compared with the 6-week convalescence associated with the traditional abdominal approach. The laparoscopic approach also appeared to be considerably less painful, as judged by the quantity of opiate analgesic required. Remarkably, neither group suffered a complication of any kind.

The work reported above was performed by very experienced laparoscopic surgeons and was still associated with some serious and possibly life-threatening complications. The more ambitious and technically difficult the procedure to be attempted, the more likely it is that serious complications will occur. Those who have avoided major problems during laparoscopic sterilization procedures should not assume that they have a technique that is good enough to avoid the increased dangers inevitably associated with more advanced procedures. The authors are aware of the many complications which have occurred and the remainder of this chapter will systematically review the complications which can, and therefore undoubtedly will, occur. We also suggest techniques to manage such complications. It is of the utmost importance that we ensure that these 'minimally invasive' techniques remain truly minimally invasive.

Veress needle- and trocar-induced vascular and viscus injury can give rise to life-threatening complications. Inadvertent traumatic perforation of the bowel or large blood-vessels during initial trocar insertion may happen even when perfect technique has been employed. We believe that to some extent this complication is beyond the control of the surgeon, for this stage of the operation is inevitably blind and involves the forceful thrusting of a sharp instrument through the abdominal wall. One quarter of all Canadian gynaecologists surveyed had experienced at least one case of sharp trocar or needle injury. One-half of these required a subsequent laparotomy to treat the complication.

Vessel injury

Injury to the aorta or iliac arteries will usually be immediately obvious with dramatic pumping of blood from the damaged vessel. This problem obviously requires immediate laparotomy to repair the damage. More insidious bleeding from a damaged vein, particularly if it leaks into the retroperitoneal space, may result in severe or fatal loss, which may not be diagnosed at the time of the initial laparoscopy. Even large-diameter veins may not bleed when they are tamponaded by the 10−15 mmHg pressure produced by the insufflation of the CO_2 distension gas. The venous pressure is reduced in the Trendelenberg position and an enlarging retroperitoneal haematoma may tamponade the damaged vessel for a time. When the pneumatoperitoneum is released at the end of the procedure, these pressure levels return to normal and major bleeding, with vascular collapse and hypovolaemic shock, can then occur. To avoid this tragedy, the course of the major vessels should be carefully inspected at the start and again at the completion of the endoscopic procedure. Any defect in the peritoneum overlying a vessel should be inspected with care. A small round defect will have been produced by the Veress needle, whilst a triangular defect indicates that the damage has been inflicted with the trocar. Trocar injuries always demand full exploration but the smaller lesions produced by the protected end of a Veress needle may be occluded spontaneously and consideration should be given to managing such a lesion expectantly.

If a haematoma is defined, the peritoneum overlying it should be opened, either with the scissors or with a suitable laser. The haematoma should then be broken up by alternating suction and irrigation with an aquadissector; the area is then cleaned and the bleeding point defined. Small-vessel bleeding may be controlled with electrosurgical desiccation and larger, isolated vessel deficiencies may be occluded with titanium clips or endoloops. If the haematoma continues to expand or the bleeding cannot be easily controlled by these measures, there must be no further delay to open laparotomy repair of the vessel, preferably with the help of a vascular surgeon. Bleeding can usually be controlled until skilled help arrives by a combination of compression to the vessel and isolating the bleeding area with vascular tourniquets of rubber or Dacron tape.

Epigastric vessels

Injury to the deep epigastric vessels can be avoided by inserting the secondary puncture trocars laterally to them. This can be done under direct vision, for, as we have previously described, we do not think that transillumination is a reliable way of locating these vessels. The deep epigastric artery arises from the external iliac artery, just distal to the bifurcation of the femoral artery. The vessel is associated with two veins, the venae comitantes, which lie either side of and immediately below the artery. They lie in the medial peritoneal fold of the internal inguinal ring, where the round ligament curls around the vessels as it enters the inguinal canal. Superficial epigastric vessels are, however, noted by transillumination and we recommend that both direct observation with the laparoscope and transillumination should be performed prior to choosing the site for secondary puncture. The deep epigastric vessels lie beneath the lateral margin of the rectus muscle, so that lateral insertion should also avoid muscle bleeding.

Should these precautions fail to prevent bleeding at the second puncture site, rotating the trocar sleeve through 360° will often produce sufficient vessel tamponade to arrest the flow and, if pressure is then applied to that spot for a few minutes, bleeding may be controlled. If the bleeding persists, the trocar sleeve should be left in position and on no account be removed. Long Kleppinger bipolar forceps may be introduced down the operating channel of the laparoscope and used to desiccate vessels above the peritoneum, both distally and proximally to the trocar site. If a haematoma is present, it should be opened and evacuated with alternating suction and irrigation until a clear effluent is obtained.

Another method of controlling haemorrhage at this site is by inserting a Foley catheter through the second-puncture trocar sleeve. The balloon is inflated and then traction is applied to the external portion of the catheter to maintain an effective tamponade. The tamponade may be maintained by placing a haemostat clamp across the catheter at skin level.

Vessels in the middle of the thickness of the abdominal wall may best be controlled by inserting large, hand-held, curved needles through the whole thickness of the abdominal wall. The intra-abdominal part of the loop can be completed under laparoscopic observation and sutures should be inserted cephalad and caudally to the trocar sleeve.

Ovarian and uterine vessel bleeding

Any of the methods described in the previous chapters to secure these vessels may also be used to arrest secondary haemorrhage or unintended damage. Individual clips, sutures and bipolar desiccation may all be tried. The collateral circulation is adequate and ligation of one of these vessels never results in major ischaemic changes.

Gastrointestinal injuries

Gastrointestinal injuries are a fairly common complication of laparoscopic surgery. Many of these may be corrected laparoscopically if the surgeon is prepared for them.

Stomach

The routine use of an orogastric tube will ensure that the stomach is empty and thereby greatly reduce the risk of perforation of this structure. If the primary trocar inadvertently enters the stomach and a percutaneous gastroscopy results, the defect can be closed by laparoscopically placing a purse-string suture in the seromuscular layer surrounding the defect. A nasogastric tube should be left in place for 2 days.

Bowel

Trocar insertion injuries

Perforation of the large and small bowel tends to occur during insertion of either the primary trocar or the Veress needle. Injury by the Veress needle is probably more common than is diagnosed for it is often not serious and may go unrecognized. Veress-needle injuries typically occur when loops of intestine are adherent to the anterior abdominal wall and the perforation seals off promptly. Expectant management is appropriate here and laparotomy is seldom required. Air insufflation into an intestinal loop was reported eight times in 500 procedures [3]. The most useful diagnostic sign is the presence of the characteristic faecal smell.

Injury with the primary trocar is more of a major problem. It is essential to diagnose this complication at the time of the laparoscopy. Delay in diagnosis leads to the development of peritonitis, which is often fatal if unrecognized for too long. The most dangerous situation is when a loop of bowel (usually transverse colon) is firmly adherent to the abdominal wall. The trocar may pass completely through the full thickness of the bowel, which may then remain transfixed by the sleeve through the whole of the procedure. The accident will not be noticed unless the operator routinely examines the contents of the entire abdominal cavity. If such a perforation is suspected, the trocar sleeve and the laparoscope should be slowly removed whilst the cavity is inspected; the perforated bowel, its lumen and its contents will then come into view.

If the surgeon is skilled at laparoscopic suturing, the defect may be closed in this manner or by using an Endo GIA 30 multifire stapling system. For most surgeons, however, repair via an open minilaparotomy incision is recommended. Colostomy is seldom indicated in this situation. The perforation may go through multiple loops of bowel and, particularly if the lesion is in the small bowel, it is often helpful to leave the trocar *in situ* until everything is ready for the repair so that the site of the damage can be conveniently marked.

Small-bowel perforation most commonly occurs during the insertion of the trocars in patients with extensive small-bowel adhesions. Usually the perforation ·is not recognized until later in the procedure, after omental and small-bowel adhesions are freed from the anterior abdominal wall. If such adhesions are not divided, the perforation may not be recognized at all. If multiple adhesions are anticipated, the primary puncture may be made at a higher site, such as the left costal margin in the midclavicular line. After establishing a pneumatoperitoneum from this site, a 5-mm telescope can be inserted and a panoramic view of the whole cavity obtained. Adhesions can then be taken down around the umbilicus and, when this area is clear, the more conventional portal can again be used.

Following recognition of a small-bowel perforation, it can be repaired laparoscopically. The defect should be closed transversely with interrupted 3−0 Vicryl, silk or PDS on a taper SH needle and tied either extracorporeally with a knot-pusher or intracorporeally. The integrity of the repair may be tested by instilling sterile milk into the bowel lumen prior to closing the last suture. Leakage from the suture line and any other occult perforations may be demonstrated in this way.

Bowel injuries occurring during dissection

Injury during surgery occurs most often at the level of the rectosigmoid. Detection and careful inspection of the lesion are again the most important steps to take. Superficial lesions can be measured by careful postoperative observation. Defects involving the full thickness of the wall require surgical repair by an experienced surgeon, either laparoscopically or by laparotomy. Laparoscopically, stay sutures of 3−0 silk, PDS or Vicryl are placed at the transverse angles of the defect and brought out through the lower-quadrant trocar sleeves, which are reinserted into the cavity over the stay sutures. The defect is then closed with interrupted sutures. The integrity of the repair can be determined by inserting a Foley catheter up the rectum and distending the 30-ml balloon. Betadine solution can then be injected above the balloon and the suture line observed. An underwater examination is done and any leaking areas are reinforced. Resection of sections of damaged bowel, with or without colostomy, should be considered but is rarely indicated.

Superficial thermal injuries to bowel noted during surgery can be treated prophylactically with a laparoscopically placed purse-string suture. This should be placed beyond the thermally affected tissue.

Delayed bowel injury

Bowel injury is usually diagnosed late either because the original injury was not detected at the time of surgery or because the bowel sustained thermal damage from any source which led to a delayed necrosis and subsequent perforation. Less frequently, delayed injuries can occur from perforation of a mechanically devitalized bowel or following mesenteric thrombosis. With a traumatic perforation the symptoms usually present within 24−48 hours of surgery. Perforation secondary to thermal injury does not present until 4−10 days later.

Open laparotomy is required for these cases. The gross appearances of the lesion are similar, whether the cause was traumatic or thermal. There is characteristically a perforation surrounded by a white area of necrosis. The histological appearances, however, are quite different following the two types of trauma. Following thermal burns there is featureless dead amorphous tissue surrounding the perforation without any polymorphonuclear infiltration, whereas following traumatic puncture injury there is abundant and rapid capillary ingrowth with white cell infiltration and fibrin deposition at the site of the injury [4].

If a perforation occurs in a patient with an unprepared bowel and substantial faecal contamination results, laparotomy, repair and extensive peritoneal toilet are indicated. If significant faecal contamination has not occurred, laparoscopic repair followed by copious irrigation until the effluent is quite clear should be satisfactory.

For many years colostomy was recommended for any traumatic bowel injury. In 1951, however, Woodhall and Ochesner [5] reported that the mortality rate for patients with traumatic bowel injury fell from 23% to 9% when primary closure replaced initial colostomy as the randomized management protocol. Morbidity was 10 times higher and the hospital stay 6 days longer when a colostomy was routinely performed. Similar results were found by George *et al.* [6] and Burch *et al.* [7]. There are therefore few data to support the routine performance of a colostomy as a part of the routine management of laparoscopically produced bowel injuries.

Bladder injuries

The bladder may be damaged during insertion of a secondary trocar or during dissection and reflection from the anterior surface of the uterus. A sinister bubbling of CO_2 down the indwelling catheter is indicative of this complication, as is the failure of the bladder to fill during a prolonged procedure. As with other complications, the most important part in the management of this problem is the early recognition of the true state of affairs. If a perforation is found, a Foley's catheter should be left in the bladder for at least 7 days and prophylactic antibiotics commenced. The defect may be closed by inserting a figure-of-eight suture through the bladder musculature and then a second suture should be used to close the overlying peritoneum. The integrity of this repair can be determined by instilling into the bladder a weak solution of methylene blue or other dye.

Postoperative urinary retention

The operation may be prolonged and large volumes of irrigating fluid may have been absorbed. Postoperative fluid retention may occur and is best prevented by leaving an indwelling Foley's catheter *in situ* for a few hours until the patient is completely awake. If spontaneous voiding does not occur within 3 hours of removal of the catheter, a further straight catheterization should be performed. The simultaneous administration of an appropriate anticholinergic drug may also be helpful in preventing urinary retention.

The ureter

The ureter is particularly vulnerable during laparoscopic hysterectomy, for it lies in close proximity to the major vessels to be ligated during the procedure. It forms the posterior boundary of the ovarian fossa at the pelvic brim and then runs medially and forward to the lateral aspect of the cervix. At the level of the ureteric canal, the ureter runs parallel to and then passes beneath the uterine artery. In these two sites the ureter may be inadvertently damaged or occluded. Sutures and clips may be misapplied, as it is often difficult to be certain of the ureter's position unless it has previously been completely dissected. Application of the Endo GIA 30 clips may be particularly dangerous, especially in the area of the ureteric canal, for these instruments are quite wide and straight and it is often difficult to correctly align them with the uterine artery and at the same time ensure that the ureter is free of the tips. For this reason, the authors do not recommend the use of Endo GIA 30 staples for occlusion of the uterine artery. Application of electrosurgical or laser energy may spread and produce unintended thermal damage, which can lead to subsequent ureteral narrowing and hydroureter.

If the surgeon is suspicious about the integrity of the ureter during the procedure, 5 ml of indigo carmine solution can be injected intravenously. This will be excreted in the urine within 5−10 minutes of injection. Any patient with postoperative flank or pelvic pain should have an intravenous urogram performed.

Hernia

Failure to close the fascial defects from incisions greater than 7 mm can lead to incisional hernia of the anterior abdominal wall. With such a size of incision, the fascia should be separated and exposed with the help of adequate illumination and skin hooks and the incision should be repaired in layers.

Infection

Intra-abdominal infection can be reduced by meticulous haemostasis and removing all blood clot from the cavity. Reich strongly recommends the underwater inspection of all vascular pedicles and careful occlusion of all bleeders. The painstaking removal of all blood clots takes away any possible focus where infection could begin.

Umbilical incision infection can be minimized by carefully cleaning the site prior to the initial incision and burying the knots beneath the deep fascia. Lower-quadrant incision infection is very rare and Harry Reich has only encountered one rectus muscle infection requiring drainage in over 2000 procedures.

Fluid overload

Fluid overload may occur if large volumes of irrigating fluid are used during lengthy procedures. It is important, therefore, to use physiologically compatible fluids such as Ringer's lactate or normal saline during these procedures. Absorption is from the peritoneal surfaces and excretion is chiefly through the kidneys, although some fluid may be lost through loosely approximated skin incisions. Pulmonary oedema can occur in these circumstances and Reich has reported an incidence of four in a series of 1000 women exposed to vigorous peritoneal lavage.

Subcutaneous emphysema and oedema

Gas or fluid may accumulate in the tissues of the abdominal wall. Manipulation of instruments often loosens the parietal peritoneum surrounding their portal of exit into the peritoneal cavity. CO_2 can then track up the loose areolar tissue of the body. The direction in which this gas flows is gravity-dependent and, if the gas enters the tissues while the patient is in a steep Trendelenberg position, it often finishes up in the shoulder and fascial regions, but vulval and upper thigh accumulations have also been noted. Subcutaneous emphysema produces characteristic crepitations which subside within a few hours. Fluid may follow a similar track and produce subcutaneous oedema.

References

1 Reich H, Decaprio J, McGlynn F. Laparoscopic hysterectomy. *J Gynae Surg* 1989; **5**: 213–216.

2 Bruhat MA, Mage G, Pouly JL, Manhes H, Canis M, Wattiez A. Laparoscopic hysterectomy. In: *Operative Laparoscopy*, pp. 217–221. McGraw-Hill, New York, 1991.

3 Vilardell F, Seres I, Marti-Vincente A. Complications of peritoneoscopy. A survey of 1455 examinations. *Gastro Endosc* 1968; **14**: 178.

4 Levey BS, Soderstrom RM, Dail DH. Bowel injuries during laparoscopy: gross anatomy and histology. *J Repro Med* 1985; **30**: 168.

5 Woodhall JP, Ochesner A. The management of perforating injuries of the colon and rectum in civilian practice. *Surgery* 1951; **29**: 305.

6 George SM, Fabian TC, Voeller GR *et al*. Primary repair of colon wounds. *Ann Surg* 1989; **209** (6): 728.

7 Burch JM, Brock JC, Gevirtzman L *et al*. The injured colon. *Ann Surg* 1986; **203** (6): 701.

14: The Future of Endoscopic Surgery: Training and Education

This book has described in some detail much of the equipment that is required to safely and effectively perform a laparoscopic hysterectomy. We have also attempted to trace the development of this equipment and have emphasized that a thorough understanding of this new equipment is an essential prerequisite for laparoscopic surgery. There have been incredible advances in electronics, optics, laser technology and instrument manufacture to facilitate operative laparoscopy. Without these technical advances laparoscopic hysterectomy would not, of course, have been possible.

New approaches, particularly those close to the core of any speciality's practice, are often resisted until they are fully evaluated, and indeed it is appropriate that this should be so. Certainly, advanced laparoscopic surgery is no exception to the rule and a recent commentary in the journal *Obstetrics and Gynecology* posed the question 'Laparoscopic surgery: advance or gimmick?' and seemed to conclude that gimmick was the more likely answer. Clearly the contributors to this book do not accept this view and, on the contrary, believe that advanced endoscopic surgery, culminating for the gynaecologist, as it does, in laparoscopic hysterectomy, represents one of the most important set of developments ever to influence operative gynaecology. It is essential that such beliefs are tested with large-scale multicentre evaluations.

This new approach and these technical advances have occurred at precisely the moment when there has also developed a patient-led demand for less invasive surgery. Whilst doctors ponder the value of these procedures, patients appear to be in less doubt. They request and, in some cases, even demand surgery which produces the minimum of scarring and morbidity. Who can blame them, for which of us, given a choice, would choose a procedure which involves an 8-inch abdominal scar when this might be avoided? It is the abdominal incision which causes much of the pain associated with major surgery. Avoiding this large incision will reduce the need for opiate analgesics, which are otherwise inevitably required. These medications then inevitably cause nausea and drowsiness and confine the patient to bed. This pain–analgesic cycle prolongs the time spent in hospital and also appears to prolong the recovery period. It is now clear that the pain–analgesic–drowsiness syndrome many had assumed was an essential part of any postoperative phase is principally a reflection of the length of the abdominal incision. A large incision produces much pain which thereby prolongs convalescence. Conversely, it has been demonstrated that smaller incisions are associated with less pain, less need for opiates, less nausea and drowsiness and quicker recovery times. Postoperative symptoms are more related to the length of the incision than the length of the operative procedure or what happened under the incision. Thanks to the excellence of modern anaesthetic techniques, many patients who have had operations lasting 3—6 hours are still fit to leave hospital within 24 hours of surgery.

The laparoscopic approach also reduces the amount of tissue handling that occurs and totally prevents the peritoneal drying which may contribute to the bowel dysfunction and 'wind' so commonly seen after open laparotomy. The brilliant magnified view obtained at laparoscopy may also allow more effective haemostasis to be achieved and efficient suction—irrigation can remove all traces of debris and blood clot and reduces the risk of postoperative infection.

The excellence of the results reported here, with a morbidity rate of 6% and a mean hospital stay of less than 2 days, poses a challenge to those who continue to advocate open surgery. How can they continue to justify abdominal hysterectomy, which is more disfiguring, more painful, associated with a longer recovery time and more complications and ultimately more expensive than the laparoscopic alternative?

The desire of patients and their relatives to be out of hospital as rapidly as possible is shared by governments and health-funding authorities throughout the world. They are all increasingly looking for value for the 'health dollar'. They can readily appreciate that procedures which are effective and command patient confidence and yet dramatically reduce costs by reducing both hospital costs and social supporting costs of surgery are politically and economically very attractive.

Health-funding authorities must realize that they will not achieve the benefits of minimally invasive endoscopic surgery on the cheap. Good results cannot be achieved without a comprehensive range of appropriate equipment. Good results will also require extensive training of all grades of staff involved in the programme. The surgeon must not only have available a full range of equipment but also ensure that he/she and his/her support staff are fully familiar with and comfortable with the use of that equipment. Above all, he/she must have adapted to the philosophy of minimally invasive surgery, with its emphasis on restricting portals of access and of conserving all tissue which is not dysfunctional or diseased.

The results reported in Chapter 13 were achieved by some of the most experienced laparoscopic surgeons in the world. Even they experienced major complications, including damage to the bladder, the ureter, the bowel and major blood-vessels. Hysterectomy, no matter by what technique it is performed, is a major and potentially dangerous operation. Most gynaecologists were taught to perform abdominal and vaginal hysterectomies in the traditional apprentice fashion by learning the principles of the procedure, observing then assisting then operating under supervision and finally operating 'solo'. The ability to safely perform abdominal and vaginal hysterectomies is an important mile-stone in the surgical training of a gynaecologist.

Who, however, is to train the new laparoscopic hysterectomist? Hysterectomy is the core operation of gynaecology, central to the practice of gynaecology, and the laparoscopic approaches have come uninvited into the lives of many who have spent years becoming expert and skilled at a procedure which may no longer be in demand. Does such a gynaecologist need retraining and, if so, how and by whom?

Almost every gynaecologist can perform diagnostic and simple operative procedures. In the minds of many, particularly those who have achieved eminence because of their excellence at open surgery, the transition to 'advanced laparoscopic surgery' is minimal and requires little or no specialized training. Doctors unfamiliar with videolaparo-scopy, however, may have problems performing a three-dimensional operation from a two-dimensional screen. All surgeons should become familiar with only one or two new pieces of equipment at a time and should steadily progress from the simplest to the more complex procedures.

There are as yet no absolute guidelines for appropriate training and accreditation in gynaecological endoscopic surgery, but it is suggested that the essential starting-point is competence at the standard open procedures. This is important in order to ensure that only suitable cases are selected for the endoscopic procedure and that the surgeon has the ability to cope with any complications that may occur. The next recommended step is to attend an accredited course. An ideal course should be specially designed for advanced laparoscopic surgery and should include didactic material about the physical principles of the equipment, particularly lasers and electrosurgical equipment. Safety factors must be extensively discussed. Then practical aspects of the procedures, including indications, contraindications and complications, should be considered. There should be a 'hands-on' element. In the UK this can only be with trainers and inanimate material but in the US and many parts of continental Europe this stage of the work can include operations on anaesthetized animals. It is ironic and unaccept-able that in the UK it is easier to practise new surgical techniques on patients than on animals. It is certainly logical to move the hand–eye co-ordination practice from bench trainers with inanimate material to appropriate animal models before patients. The course should then illustrate actual procedures, first with tightly edited videos, then with closed-circuit transmission and finally in the operating room. Once in the OR, the gynaecologist must be aware of all the equipment used, including the setting up and safety features of each item. He/she should study the roles of the nurses and laser operatives and become familiar with the procedures undertaken at first hand. It is recommended that the trainee laparoscopist then assists at 5–10 complex procedures under the personal supervision of a trained endoscopist and then attempts a further 5—10 cases with an experienced laparoscopist in attendance before undertaking such procedures on his/her own.

Whether such recommendations become the basis for formal accreditation/credentials or just informal guidelines for good practice will depend on local customs and practices. It is essential for the well-being of the patient and the future of endoscopic surgery that this new approach is not discredited by inexperienced surgeons (in laparoscopy, not general experience) attempting too much too soon. No degree of eminence at open surgery exempts the doctor from the need to gain appropriate endoscopic training.

If introduced slowly and with care and if complemented by further contributions from the engineers and scientists, it is possible that most gynaecological operations will be performed laparoscopically. The authors believe that endoscopically and classically trained gynaecologists will be able to offer to their patients the widest possible choice of therapeutic options and it is increasingly probable that they will choose the laparoscopic hysterectomy and laparoscopic-assisted vaginal hysterectomy options.

Index